DATE DUE

Sex Drive, Healthy You

WHAT YOUR LIBIDO REVEALS
ABOUT YOUR LIFE

Healthy Sex Drive, Healthy You

WHAT YOUR LIBIDO REVEALS ABOUT YOUR LIFE

DIANA HOPPE, M.D.

Foreword by Carolle Jean-Murat, M.D.

HEALTH REFLECTIONS PRESS

Encinitas, California

2010

Publisher's Cataloging in Publication Data

Hoppe, Diana.
Healthy sex drive, healthy you : what your libido reveals about your
life / Diana Hoppe ; f oreword by Carolle Jean-Murat.—Encinitas,
Calif. : Health Reflections Press, 2010.

p. ; cm.
ISBN: 978-0-9825411-0-4
Includes bibliographical references and index.

1. Women–Sexual behavior. 2. Sex–Health aspects.
3. Women–Health and hygiene. 4. Sex (Psychology) I. Title.

HQ29 .H67 2010 2009936189
306.7/082– dc22 1004

ISBN 978-0-9825411-0-4

Publisher: Health Reflections Press
P.O. Box 231187
Encinitas, CA 92023

A BookStudio Production, www.bookstudiobooks.com
Produced by Karla Olson

Copyedited by Lisa Wolff

Book design by Claudine Mansour Design, www.claudinemansour.com

www.DrDianaHoppe.com

TABLE OF CONTENTS

ACKNOWLEDGMENTS

As an OB/Gyn, I have accompanied many women through their pregnancies, guiding them through the nine months of gestation to the amazing joy at the time of delivery. Writing this book has been much like a pregnancy, although the gestation period was more like three-and-a-half years not 40 weeks!

Through this time, many wonderful people have helped me "gestate" and "deliver" this literary creation. I would first like to thank the person who truly made this book possible, my literary agent, Bettie Youngs, PhD. Without your unwavering support and true belief in this book, it would never have been "born." The terrific editing of Susan Heim, Elisabeth Rinaldi, and Donna DiBenedetto helped make my scientific jargon more accessible, engaging, and entertaining. I thank Karla Olson for her skillful guidance in connecting me with amazing people and resources to make this book the best it could be. Graphic designer Claudine Mansour's talent and creativity helped me find the perfect cover and interior design—slightly sexy but not too "cosmo." I would like to thank my dear friends, Carolyn Edwards, Jennifer Tran, and Tole Markinkovic, who patiently listened to me over the years and supported me with their wisdom and faith. I am grateful to my loving partner, Scott Escher, who has championed me through this endeavor and made me understand why this book is valuable and necessary to both women *and* men. Lastly, I wish to thank my patients, because of their honesty, candor, and persistence in asking, "Dr. Hoppe, what can I do for my libido?", this book was conceived, developed, and finally born—weighing 7 oz., measuring 6 inches by 9 inches, and screaming to be read. Thank you!

FOREWORD

Born and raised in Haiti, I had the privilege to live and be educated in the best universities in four different countries including the United States. For the past three decades, I have worked with women from all over the world and from all walks of life, as a board-certified gynecologist, an intuitive consultant, and, lately, offering one-on-one retreats to women. Thousands have trusted me as their gynecologist, surgeon, healer, confidante, sister/friend, and intuitive counselor, with excellent results. Many had ample time to connect and were given the opportunity to share their innermost secrets with me.

One of the most common sexual complaints among women is a lack of desire for sex. Yet despite its pervasiveness, it is a problem that many women suffer in silence. Though we live in a time of supposedly open communication about sex, a survey of adults 25 and older revealed that 71 percent believed their health-care provider would dismiss any sexual concerns they might bring up, and about 68 percent avoided discussing sexual problems because they were embarrassed.

Even if a woman is not reluctant to voice sexual complaints to her health-care provider, she may be confronted with someone who is ill-equipped or simply too busy to properly evaluate and treat these problems. A successful treatment approach requires a complete understanding of the psychology and physiology of female sexual response, as well as the time to sort out what is going on in a woman's life as a whole. Although low libido has been associated with hormone imbalance, other factors, especially stress, often lead to physical and mental symptoms, including sexual ones.

Many women, then, simply do not know where to turn for help with sexual problems. They hunger for trustworthy information that is clear and easy to understand. At last, there is a book that fulfills this need: Dr. Hoppe's *Healthy Sex Drive, Healthy You: What Your Libido Reveals about Your Life.*

Dr. Hoppe has written a remarkably practical and informative guide to excellent sexual health for women. Woven into the tapestry of her message is the expert knowledge of a gynecologist, a woman, and a researcher, along with common sense and the wisdom gained from many years of experience.

This book is much more than a guide to better sexual health, however. It beautifully integrates mind and body, taking a holistic approach to sexual problems. Good sexual health is treated as part of overall good health, and Dr. Hoppe provides specific, practical advice for dealing with common problems that may affect a woman's sex life, as well as guidance on how to improve relationships with both her intimate partner and her health-care provider. This approach makes the book much more comprehensive than other sources.

The information contained in this book is an invaluable aid to helping women overcome the obstacles standing between them and sexual fulfillment. Even women who have never before achieved a satisfying and fulfilling sexual life can do so, with the help of Dr. Hoppe's extraordinary book.

—CAROLLE JEAN-MURAT, M.D., F.A.C.O.G.,
author of the best-selling and award-winning
Menopause Made Easy and
*Mind, Body, Soul & Money: Putting Your Life
in Balance*

INTRODUCTION

Women are absolutely amazing. Somehow, we dedicate 100 percent of our hearts and minds to our families, our work, and our community. We are organized, smart, nurturing, and generous. We are intensely well informed about how to manage our finances, cook chicken in 365 different ways, write a brilliant résumé, and be the best parent who ever lived. What we tend to overlook, however, is becoming as well informed as possible about our private concerns: our mental, physical, and sexual health. You have taken an important step in empowering yourself to take control of your health and happiness by reading this book.

According to a National Health and Social Survey, approximately 43 percent of American women—including those in their early childbearing years—have some form of "sexual dysfunction," the majority suffering from *decreased* sexual desire. Yes, almost half of American women—many in the prime of their sexual lives—would rather choose sleep, a good book, or a soothing bath over having sex with their partner. What about you? Take a close look at how you are living your life. Are you putting your physical, emotional, and spiritual needs last?

By keenly assessing the choices you make, you can find the strength and power to live a more satisfying, fulfilling life. As a woman, it's important to become aware of the highly significant connection between your libido and your quality of life. A pleasurable sex life spills over into the rest of your life. In fact, sex is good for your health—it can lead to a longer life span, less stress and depression, a healthier immune system, as well as more loving relationships, a greater sense of self-esteem, more enjoyment and satisfaction from life, and a feeling of recaptured sexual vigor—all things that women strive for.

Fortunately, signs indicate that women aren't ready to accept a passionless life. Certainly this sentiment is at the heart of what I hear from women! In Pfizer's 2007 Global Study of Sexual Attitudes and Behaviors, 64 percent of women (ages 40 to 80) in 28 countries felt that sex was an important part of their lives, and that physical and sexual satisfaction were highly correlated with feeling healthy and happy. Nearly 70 percent of those who described their health as "excellent" also reported that their physical relationship with their partner was extremely pleasurable. A similar trend exists between emotional satisfaction and health. Those who described their sex lives as less than satisfying expressed an interest in wanting to reverse this condition—to "recharge their libido." Clearly, women are frustrated and want to regain control of their lives—both in and out of the bedroom.

From the beginning of my medical training until today, I have always had an interest in women's health issues, especially sexual desire. Through personally conducting this research, my passion for helping women find ways to make their lives more exciting and fulfilling has magnified. The phenomenal connection between libido and general well-being, in emotional, physical, and spiritual realms, is my inspiration to continue researching and exploring.

The latest research and techniques presented in this book can help you take control of your health and relationships. This book will cover new information, such as the most recent brain research targeting specific areas of brain function (especially those impacting sex or orgasm), and new drugs aimed at tackling the core issues affecting women's libido. Examples include:

- By improving your intimate relationship, you can decrease your risk for heart disease. Recent studies have shown a connection between marriages marked by negativity, such as conflict and adverse exchanges, and an increase in the risk of heart disease (by 34 percent), even after factoring in other contributors to heart disease.

- Switching from a high-fat, refined-carbohydrate diet to one containing more organic, raw, and unprocessed foods has been shown to be beneficial in regulating women's hormones. Fatty tissue contains an enzyme that converts adrenal steroids into estrogen. The more fat you take in and the higher amount of body fat you have, the higher the rate of conversion of estrogen in your body, resulting in overall higher estrogen levels. Decreasing the amount of fat in your diet can therefore help in better balancing your hormone levels, as well as dramatically decreasing your risk for heart disease.

■ Women are known as the ultimate multitaskers. But this seemingly positive ability can actually decrease your desire for physical intimacy, and negatively impact your emotional and physical health. Studies have found that multitasking increases the level of stress-related hormones (such as cortisol and adrenaline) and wears down your system through biochemical friction, causing premature aging. In the short term, the confusion, fatigue, and chaos resulting from multitasking merely hampers your ability to focus and analyze; in the long term, however, it may cause your health to atrophy, in addition to killing libido.

■ Unfortunately, the "little blue pill" (Viagra) that often works so well in enhancing sexual performance for men does not produce the same benefits in women. Presently, a deluge of pharmaceutical companies is working on finding the new female libido-enhancing drug, possibly the new "pink Viagra." This search for the next Holy Grail has led to the development of pills that act on certain neurotransmitters (dopamine and serotonin), testosterone patches, and clitoral pumps—all of which can help jump-start your libido. Some over-the-counter products—including dehydroepiandrosterone (DHEA) and Argin-Max, an amino acid L-arginine supplement—may also produce increased sexual desire and satisfaction in users.

In 20 years of practice, I've successfully helped thousands of women restore (and/or balance) their libido. I have learned that helping a woman achieve better sexual health is not only possible, but easily attainable! Of course, you can find plenty of advice—most of it unproven—about improving sexual satisfaction. And men certainly have an edge in the sex department with the discovery of Viagra! But a pill or a new negligee isn't the answer for women. What is new and fresh about the solutions in this book is the simplicity of moving toward a better sense of well-being. Throughout this book, I'll provide the "prescription" you need to get things right in your head and in your life, so you can get it right in the bedroom. If you have been frustrated with the roller coaster you've been riding in your sexual life, know that it can be "fixed."

Are you ready to really listen to your libido? A critical objective of this book is to *give you permission* to be sexy and sexual! You deserve to experience the fullness and joy of great sexual intimacy! But in order to do so, you must be informed. Understand your body and your brain and the processes that govern sexuality, as well as those that create a reluctance to enjoy intimacy. When you (and your partner) have the facts and the language to express this important element of your life, you can communicate more effectively. This candid communication can not only save your relationship, but also prove to get the sexual juices flowing. The choice to be happy and healthy sexually is within your control!

—*Diana Hoppe, M.D.*

Healthy Sex Drive, Healthy You

WHAT YOUR LIBIDO REVEALS
ABOUT YOUR LIFE

CHAPTER 1

Eight Reasons Why Sex Is Good for You—and Why It's Wise to Make Time for Sexual Intimacy

"Make love when you can. It's good for you."
—Kurt Vonnegut, Jr.

Joanne, a 42-year-old account executive, was like a good many of my patients. In my office for her annual physical exam, she complained of an overall lack of energy. She revealed that she had been under a lot of stress at work, and it was making her feel down. She thought she "looked tired and old" when she looked at herself in the mirror. After inquiring further about her symptoms, I recommended more rest and some dietary changes. I also gave some general counseling on how she could manage her stress, and then I requested we run some blood work to rule out any medical conditions such as a sluggish thyroid. When I concluded all of this testing, I asked her, "So, Joanne, how is your libido?"

Surprised at my inquiry, Joanne replied, "Well, if you're asking about my sex life, I'd say it's almost nonexistent. Why do you ask?"

I understood her astonishment. Many people don't stop to consider that their sex lives may be a factor in their overall health. I informed Joanne that though we don't always associate libido with wellness, it does have a say in our physical and emotional wellness.

"I'm just so tired these days—my interest in sex has all but disappeared."

"Perhaps that's part of the reason why you're feeling so down and tired," I said. "Your husband might be pleased to know that I often prescribe more sex to my patients who are under a lot of stress and experiencing the physical consequences of it. Some studies even show that having sex may actually help alleviate the symptoms of stress, improve your health, and help you live longer. Of course it helps to make time for enough sleep so you're not feeling so tired and to eat a healthy diet. I'd just like to see you add a goal to this regimen of having sex two to three times per week. Try this for three months, and then I'd like to reevaluate your symptoms."

"I used to like having sex," Joanne mused and then added, "and I really do miss the intimacy it added to my marriage. Well, I'm sure my husband will be thrilled with your diagnosis and suggested remedy!"

What Exactly Is "Sex"?

Although it seems like it is obvious, I've learned in my practice that every person defines sex differently. For the purposes of this book, I consider all of the following "sex":

Sexual Activity: Includes caressing, hugging, foreplay, masturbation, and vaginal intercourse

Sexual Intercourse: Defined as penile penetration (entry) into the vagina

Sexual Stimulation: Includes foreplay with partner, self-stimulation (masturbation), and sexual fantasy

Top Eight Health Benefits of Physical Intimacy

Prescribe sex to a patient to improve her physical health? My prescription may have surprised you, too. The act of sex, however, has numerous health benefits for both men and women. Knowing these benefits may prompt you to evaluate your own libido and learn how a healthy sex life can help your overall health as well. In this chapter, I will suggest ways in which you may make such an assessment.

The following are eight reasons for creating and maintaining a healthy sex life:

1. **Sex promotes longevity.** Is this a reason to spruce up your sex life, or what!? And, imagine telling your partner you have a way to add years to your lives! According to Dr. David Weeks, a clinical neuropsychologist and author of *Secrets of the Superyoung,* sex actually slows the aging process.[1] He studied 3,500 people ranging in age from 18 to 102. The results? Those individuals who engaged in sex on a regular basis appeared to be much younger than their chronological age. They had fewer wrinkles, stood taller with better posture, had better tone to their skin color, and seemed to have a

more youthful and lighthearted general attitude and demeanor.

Why is this so? One reason may be related to the importance of touch. Dr. Teresa Crenshaw defines the power of touch as "Vitamin T."[2] Through caressing, hugging, stroking, and cuddling, the body releases a chain reaction of chemicals that sends a signal to your brain that what you are experiencing is pleasurable, nurturing, and good.

That touch is critical to good health is further documented. In the 1930s, Dr. Rene Spitz, attending physician at a number of baby nurseries, noticed that illness and mortality rates were much higher in certain nurseries as compared to others.[3] His observations and experiments discovered that children were becoming ill and dying despite good hygiene and nutrition. Why? The infants needed more physical contact from the attending staff. He solved the problem by hiring "grandmothers" to come to the nurseries to hold, caress, and cuddle the children. The illness and mortality rates declined rapidly.

Researchers at Miami's Touch Research Institute have similar findings.[4] They found that premature infants who received three massages a day over 10 days gained 47 percent more weight than their premature counterparts who did not receive such treatment. It seems logical that the touching engaged in during sexual activity can benefit adult life spans, too.

"Sex alleviates tension. Love causes it." —WOODY ALLEN

2. Sex eases depression and alleviates stress. Imagine that! Sex as an emotional pick-me up! Not that it's a reason to use sex to get together with just anyone. But used in the right way and with the right person, sex can have both uplifting and calming effects. According to Jennifer Bass, at the Kinsey Institute for Research in Sex, Gender, and Reproduction, "The release from orgasm does much towards calming people. It helps with sleep, and that is whether we talk about solo sex or sex with a partner."[5] Many studies also show that sleep may be deeper and more restful after engaging in satisfying sexual intercourse because it allows the release of distracting thoughts and negative thinking behaviors. Engaging in sex prior to falling asleep at night also decreases instances of insomnia.

Believe it or not, male semen can also alleviate depression! According to a study conducted by the State University of New York in Albany, components found in a man's ejaculate may actually have healing qualities and may act as antidepressants.[6] Females in the study who were engaging in sex without the use of condoms had fewer signs of depression than women who used condoms or abstained from sex. "These data are consistent with the possibility that semen may antagonize depressive symptoms," the authors wrote. These antidepressive effects were noted within only a few hours of when the semen had been absorbed through the vagina into the bloodstream. According to the authors, in addition to chromosomal DNA, semen contains other essential elements: prostaglandins, zinc, calcium, potassium, fructose, and proteins. Is semen a virtual vitamin blast for your vitality? It appears so. Despite this advantage, I recommend that you do use some method of birth control if you are not wanting to get pregnant and take necessary precautions against sexually transmitted diseases, such as using condoms.

"The good thing about masturbation
is that you don't have to get dressed up for it."
— TRUMAN CAPOTE

3. Sex boosts the immune system. Who would have thought that sex might be a way to help prevent the common cold and flu by boosting your immune system's defenses? Consider this: Healthy sex increases the body's natural production of antibodies, specifically levels of immunoglobulin A (IgA), which are the first line of defense in helping to fight against widespread infectious diseases such as flu and cold viruses. It's interesting to note here that sex has added benefits for men: it increases the flow of testosterone, which strengthens bones and muscles and helps transport DHEA, a hormone important in the function of the body's immune system. During orgasm, the level of DHEA in the bloodstream increases to five times its normal circulating level. Dr. Theresa Crenshaw notes that DHEA has other benefits and may be the most powerful chemical in our personal world. Besides balancing the immune system, it improves cognition, promotes bone growth, maintains and repairs tissues, and helps to keep your skin healthy and supple.

"Nothing risqué, nothing gained." —ALEXANDER WOOLLCOTT

4. Sex improves brain health. Can't remember the last time you had sex? Having more sex can improve certain brain functions, including memory, and can also improve your sense of smell. With any form of exercise—and let's face it, sex is a form of exercise—blood flow increases. This increased circulation of blood transports oxygen-enriched blood to the hypothalamus, the center of the brain for memory and learning. Thus, memory and brain function may be increased with sexual activity.

Sex can even help your brain revitalize its sense of smell. In his article "Is Sex Necessary?" Alan Farnham notes that after sexual activity, the hormone prolactin is released from the posterior pituitary gland in the brain.[7] This causes stem cells in the brain to develop new neurons in the brain's olfactory bulb, its smell center, enhancing a person's sense of smell.

"I seem to have lost my sex drive, and I'm not quite sure
how that happened. I do know that once it was a healthy and
happy part of my relationship with my husband,
and now we're lucky if we have sex once a month."
—JANE TROYER, AGE 47

5. Sex preserves vaginal health. "Use it or lose it" is literally true. Many studies in postmenopausal women have shown that they suffer less vaginal pain and atrophy, and less thinning of the vaginal lining, when they are having consistent, regular sexual activity. Vaginal atrophy can lead to vaginal dryness and itching, as well as urinary tract infections. In women, sex increases blood flow to the vagina, keeping vaginal tissues more supple and lubricated—all of which can lead to less pain with intercourse as we age.

6. Sex is healthy for the body. Is sex better for your health than an aerobics class? We all know that exercise is good for health. It wards off illness and disease, increases our strength and stamina, and keeps us fit. But

Sex as Exercise: How Does Sex Stack Up against Other Forms of Exercise?

Sexual intercourse burns approximately 150–200 calories per half-hour. How do other forms of exercise stack up?

House cleaning:	120–150 calories/half-hour
Golf:	125–145 calories/half-hour
Dancing (rock):	130–150 calories/half-hour
Yoga:	130–200 calories/half-hour
Walking (3.5 mph):	190–230 calories/half-hour
Jogging (6 mph):	270–380 calories/half-hour

Averages based on healthy 140-pound woman and a healthy 175-pound man.[8]

sweating through an exercise class or spending an hour on the treadmill is not the only way to burn calories and stay in shape. We can have sex! Of course, the number of calories burned during sex is determined somewhat by the duration and frequency of your encounters. In general, it is estimated that 30 minutes of sex expends about 150 to 200 calories. The pulse rate of a sexually excited individual increases from 70 to 150 beats per minute, which is comparable to the efforts of a weightlifter or a brisk walker. Just one incident of sexual intercourse burns the same amount of calories as running on a treadmill for 15 minutes! So, which would you rather do?

Of course, your level of physical involvement in the act of sex (passive or active) also factors into the equation. According to Bass, "Sex is not necessarily a sport. It depends on how active you are (in general). The intensity of sexual activity depends on how physically fit a person is." But even a fairly gentle session of sex will burn calories and do so in a way you may find quite a bit more pleasurable than what the treadmill can offer!

7. Sex assists in relieving pain. Orgasm can be a powerful painkiller. Oxytocin, the bonding hormone that is released before and during orgasm, calms and soothes the body. Prior to the culminating moment of an act of love, the brain emits three to five times the usual levels of oxytocin. The release of this hormone during sex also reduces the perception of pain. According to famed sexologist and author Beverly Whipple, when women masturbate to orgasm, "the pain tolerance threshold and pain detection threshold increased significantly by 74.6 percent and 106.7 percent respectively."[9] Some studies have even concluded that due to the release of these natural opiates, sex is a powerful analgesic, elevating the pain threshold and helping to relieve the aches of conditions such as arthritis, whiplash, and headaches.

In addition, natural opiate-like hormones called endorphins are released during orgasm. Remember the concept of "runner's high"? After running a certain distance, the runner no longer feels pain as the brain releases large amounts of naturally occurring endorphins. In addition to decreasing pain, endorphins produce a spiritually elevating effect and positive perception of the environment.

"I'm not sure why my libido is suddenly so low.
All I know is that if Brad Pitt walked into the room today,
I would ask him to babysit my kids."
—PATIENT OF DR. HOPPE, AGE 37

8. Sex heals physical and emotional wounds. Engaging in sexual activity with someone you love promotes healing on all levels. It fosters physical, emotional, mental, and spiritual connections, and gives us the intimate human contact we need. The release of oxytocin, for example, assists in the physical healing of wounds. Several experiments have shown that oxytocin, by regenerating certain cells, can even help heal stubborn skin sores, as seen in diabetics.

Through intimate contact with a loving partner, emotional wounds may be healed and a closer connection with your partner can be achieved. According to Dr. Dean Ornish, author of *Love and Survival: The Scientific Basis for the Healing Power of Intimacy,* "an open heart can lead to the most joyful and ecstatic sex." His research into intimacy and its effects on health have shown that "anything that promotes feelings of love and

Intimacy, Healthy Sex, and Celibacy

The positive attributes of a healthy sex life encourage overall health and wellness. Of course, having unlimited sex with multiple partners or engaging in other risky sexual behaviors is not going to produce health benefits and will actually negate any health benefits, since this behavior can produce anxiety or fear and increases the odds of contracting a sexually transmitted disease. Thus, intimacy plays a key role in the health benefits of sex, which most often comes when you are in a satisfying, committed, and monogamous relationship.

So what do you do when you are not in such a relationship? Try giving celibacy a try. Surprised?

When used in a conscious way, celibacy helps you detoxify from destructive sexual behaviors such as sexual addictions. It also gives you time alone to clarify the deeper wants and needs you are looking for in a relationship. When combined with counseling, self-reflection, and spiritual practice, celibacy can also help you heal from sexual traumas. And, it can be a time to discover more about your body and learn about the joys of pleasuring yourself.

In short, it is an opportunity for you to get healthier, increasing the likelihood that you will have healthier sex when you are once again ready for a partner.

intimacy is healing. Sex is no exception, and this is the most important health benefit of sex."[10] Many people are fearful of truly loving or trusting another person. But doing so does promote deeper connections with others and also enhances sexual pleasure.

How to Keep Your Libido in Top Shape

Data and research continue to support the health benefits resulting from a committed and satisfying sex life. Awareness of these benefits may be just the motivation you need to hop into bed with your partner. A word

Frequently Asked Question...

So what is the "magic number" for how often we should have sex? Dr. Mehmet Oz, Oprah's favorite physician and frequent co-host, recently conducted a quiz in which he posed this intriguing question. He suggests 200 times a year and believes that this can reduce your physiologic age by approximately six years. Most OB/GYNs would agree with this. I'd modify this response by adding that the amount of sexual activity that you and your partner should have is really as much as *you* want. Of course, your partner is an essential contributor to making the decision of how much sex you both want to have—and this number needs to be discussed and worked out between the two of you. Over the years, this number may wax and wane. The important thing is that you and your partner are sexually intimate in a healthy emotional and physical way. Over time, this will benefit both of you greatly!

To better figure out this number, I ask my patients: If you could take away all of your stress, time restraints, hormonal fluctuations, thoughts about body image, et cetera, how often would you actually want sex with your partner? How often would your partner want sex? Are there any other types of physical or sexual intimacy that you and your partner could explore to feel more emotionally and spiritually connected? By venturing into these arenas of intimacy with an open mind and vulnerability to seek pleasure, you and your partner can honestly communicate your needs and be better able to provide each other pleasure. Eventually, you and your partner will come upon the "number" that works best for the two of you, ultimately leading to greater health, happiness, and longevity.

of caution, however: Any physical symptoms, such as severe fatigue, depression, or pelvic pain, should be thoroughly evaluated and discussed with your doctor. Also note that certain medications may decrease your ability to experience sexual benefits, or, for men, the ability to achieve erection. This subject will be discussed further in Chapter 8. When dis-

Masturbation: The Facts

Despite lingering social taboos, statistics show that approximately 94 percent of all men and 89 percent of all women masturbate on a regular basis at some point in their lives. Masturbation, or self stimulation, releases endorphins and hormones as during other forms of sexual activity. It has been shown to improve overall health as well as sleep patterns and mood and release sexual tension or frustration. You can also use masturbation as a "learning" tool—to discover then share with your partner your most erogenous areas and how to stimulate them.

cussing these issues with your physician, make sure to mention all your medications, including herbal and alternative remedies. If, like Joanne, you get a clean bill of health and still feel that not all is well, make an effort to get on a regimen of more regular sex. It just may add new vitality to your overall sense of wellness.

In order to experience a great sex life, couples need to openly communicate. Express your desires to each other and talk openly about any problems that may be causing emotional distress. A healthy physical sex life depends strongly on a strong emotional bond between couples. Perhaps the best way to get the sexual juices flowing is through "foreplay," using your heart and mind to lovingly communicate with your partner.

Six Great Ways to Fan the Flames

1. Take care of yourself. Work out, eat healthfully, and pay attention to your physical appearance. Visit your doctor and, yes, your dentist regularly. All this will make you feel better and more self-confident.

2. Schedule sex. Make time for it. Scheduling a date night may not seem very romantic, but why not give it a try? You probably schedule many other things in life, so why not set aside time for intimacy?

Frequently Asked Question...

Why is having a "good sex life" so important? If I'm not having sex, am I doing something unhealthy to my body?

It is extremely important! I believe a healthy libido is a key barometer of the quality of your overall life. Every day, new studies show that being in a happy, fulfilling relationship that is emotionally, spiritually, and physically satisfying markedly improves your health. For example, by improving the quality of your intimate relationship with your partner and by sharing positive sexual experiences, you can decrease both your and your partner's risk for heart disease. Recent studies have shown a definite connection between marriages marked by negativity, such as conflict and adverse exchanges, and an increased risk of heart disease (by 34 percent), even after factoring in other contributors to heart disease.

If you are not presently in a relationship, taking a break from sexual intimacy can help you explore what it is you really want and are looking for. On the other hand, if you are presently in a relationship that is not emotionally or sexually satisfying, you may be doing something harmful to your mind, body, and soul. Through months or years of built up resentment and denial of deserved happiness, you actually cause weakening of your immune system, making you more susceptible to certain diseases. Now is the time to look closely at your quality of life, looking at many aspects, including how you feel about your body, your communication with your partner, and the level of romance and fun you are having on a daily basis. Now is the time to make changes and start living a more fulfilling, satisfying life—both in and out of the bedroom.

3. Dress for success. A woman in lingerie, a sexy little dress, or maybe a pair of stilettos, or a man wearing a sexy black sweater, a soft silk shirt, or great-fitting jeans, feels sexy and excited for intimacy.

4. Talk about sex with your partner. Be honest about what you like and dislike. Talk about the act itself. Also, talk about love. What parts of your lover's body do you think are the sexiest? What does he do in ordinary life that turns you on? What does he do in the bedroom to turn you on? Are you drawn to his walk? Voice? Laugh? Remind each other why you are attracted to one another. Be grateful and appreciate each other.

5. Write love letters to your partner. Scent them with your personal trademark perfume. "Stamp" it with a kiss in your favorite-colored lipstick.

6. Read sexy stories to each other. Try Anaïs Nin's *Little Birds.*

Questions for Reflection

1. How would you describe the level of your libido? Are you satisfied with this level of desire?

2. What types of regular exercise do you engage in? How much time do you spend doing cardiovascular/high-intensity workouts?

3. How do you feel about your body? Is your body image interfering with your desire for sex or your performance? Are you willing to change your perception or your body? What are you willing to do to change?

4. Do you feel as if you're too tired or stressed out for sex? How many times per week or month are you actually having sex or sharing in physical intimacy?

5. Are you willing to engage in more sex to help improve your health?

6. What *physical* benefits would you like to experience from a better sex life?

7. What *emotional* benefits would you like to experience from a better sex life?

CHAPTER 2

What Is Libido— and Why Is It Erratic?

"Am I sexually active? Not really...I just lie there."
—PATIENT OF DR. HOPPE

A PATIENT OF MINE, Natalie, is a 39-year-old attorney, wife, and mother. She describes her career as demanding, but enjoys everything about it—except that it doesn't leave much time for her three-year-old or her husband, Mark. "We used to have regular date nights," she said. "That was our one-on-one alone time, and we could always count on the evening ending in lovemaking. But we've had to forgo that time together because our little son needs that night with us as much as Mark and I need time alone. The thing is, now that we focus on being a family, we've gotten— or, at least, I've gotten—out of the role of being a lover. I'm puzzled that my sex drive has dwindled so much. I used to be more interested in sex."

When Natalie realized that she and Mark hadn't had sex in three months, she grew concerned and made an appointment to see me. "Mark and I love one another very much, but I find that when he turns to me for sex, I say no, or else I rush through it to 'get it over with.' In other words, I'm going through the motions, but my body and brain aren't into it. What's going on with me?"

"It's time to listen to your libido," I told her. "It's talking to you. What do you think it's saying?"

"Libido? I don't think it's saying anything to me," she replied. "Or maybe I'm just not listening." Natalie seemed confused and defeated. "Look, there really isn't anything in my life that I can give or do more or less of, if you know what I mean. It's not like I can just wait to share a better sex life with Mark when we do manage to get away for a few days at a time. Isn't there a prescription you can write? I just want to be able to turn on my desire for sex when Mark does."

Stages in a Woman's Life and Their Effect on Libido

Menstrual cycle

Follicular phase	Desire fuels up
Ovulation	Desire is on full "go"
Luteal phase	Desire diminishes

Pregnancy	Desire fluctuates between "yes" and "no"
Postpartum	Desire dies out
Perimenopause	Desire fluctuates, but tends to be "maybe"
Menopause	Desire fluctuates between "red hot" and "NO"

Libido 101: Understanding the Basics

Natalie's concerns—and request for a prescription—are common for many women, especially those with an all-too-busy life. When I suggested to Natalie that she listen to her libido, her response indicated that she really didn't know exactly what "libido" is or how to understand it. I get the same sort of response from many of my patients. So, let's take a closer look at what "libido" really means.

Steadman's Medical Dictionary—a go-to guide for doctors—defines it as "the conscious or unconscious sexual desire; creative desire; passionate interest; or form of life force." Carl Jung, the famous Swiss psychoanalyst, referred to libido as the psychic energy from all instinctive biological—primarily reproductive—drives. In short, libido is sexual desire. And, like all forces within us, libido has its reason for being. In other words, it serves our bodies—and our lives—in important ways. Let me quickly take you through Mother Nature's basic plan for how libido functions in our lives and why.

Frequently Asked Question...

What exactly is libido, and what's the difference between sex and libido?

In general, sex is the physical act of making love, having intercourse. Sex is what got each of us here. Libido is the drive that fuels the desire to have sex. Having thoughts, fantasies, and dreams about sex are also part of libido. Sexual intimacy includes many things in addition to intercourse, including caressing, holding hands, snuggling, foreplay, and feeling "connected" to your partner. When you feel this connection, many physiological chain reactions occur in your body—hormones are rushing to different parts of your body, brain chemicals interact with one another, and even your immune system strengthens! Emotional and physical intimacy serve a definite biological function, and their connection to your overall health is real. You might be very surprised to learn how intimately connected your level of sexual desire is to your general well-being!

The Urge to Merge: Libido's Job to Get Humans to "Hook Up"

One job of our libido is to get the sexes together to govern our biology of procreation—the "urge to merge." Obviously, the function between men and women is dramatically different and, accordingly, intensity varies greatly between the sexes. In general, men tend to have stronger sex drives than women. In fact, their brains were developed to think more about sex than women. (Men have 2.5 times the size of a specific brain area devoted to sex drive in comparison to women.)

Not only do women have (generally speaking) a lesser drive for sex than do men, but for women, libido fluctuates over the course of a lifetime. It is not uncommon for a woman in her late teens or early twenties to be constantly dreaming and fantasizing about sex. But this is hardly the case at other times in her life, when sex is not only the last thing

on her mind, but may even be considered a chore or unnecessary altogether. And there are times when sex drive fluctuates within the monthly
cycle, as well as during specific life stages when the body sends cues as to
the degree of desire. In other words, there's a biology to it all.

Mother Nature's Plan

There are natural, biological reasons for the ups and downs—the fluctua-
tion—of sexual desire in women. Mother Nature very shrewdly configured
our hormones and our responses to them. She encourages increased sex
drive at certain key times that are beneficial to our species from a biological and evolutionary standpoint. These strong hormonal influences begin
at birth. When a female child is born, her ovaries contain the maximum
number of eggs she will ever have in her lifetime. In fact, at the sixth
month of development, the female fetus possesses the greatest number of
eggs and the number declines from then on. By the time of her first menstrual cycle, or period, the number of eggs has markedly decreased. The
quality of her eggs at this time, however, is at their prime, the most fertile
and chromosomally healthy. As a woman ages, her eggs are exposed to
the years of chemicals, toxins, and changes that make them less likely to
produce a chromosomally normal, viable embryo. At the time of menopause, her ovaries will no longer ovulate, or release an egg to be fertilized.
As this process occurs, a woman may experience significant emotional
and physical changes (which will be discussed later in this chapter).

So when women comment or complain about their sex drive waning
or being "on overdrive," there is a biological reason. Still, in my more
than 15 years of clinical practice as an OB/GYN, I have noticed that
in recent years, more and more of my patients complain of decreased
desire—some of them even in their late twenties, when the body is typi-
cally ruling a woman's desire to be "ON." But women of all ages want to
know how to fuel their desire so that at least it is something they control.
Understandably, this lowered sex drive is perplexing, and they want to
know why their desire for sex has dwindled. Invariably, a concerned 20-
something patient will ask, "How do I make sure I don't have something

wrong with me, like cancer?" When a woman's body isn't responding the way she wants it to, fears creep in.

A woman's emotions are further complicated by the fact that while the female sex drive is fluctuating, that isn't the case with the man in her life. She may feel as if she is less than a woman and is disappointing her mate. "My husband/partner is always in the mood, while I'm not," many women complain. These differences in sexual drive will be further explored in Chapter 4. The fact that women's and men's sex drives are vastly different poses challenging relationship issues. These are some of the questions I hear from my patients and their partners:

Women ask:

Why am I having a "sex drive crisis"?

Is the amount of sex my partner and I are having "normal"?

If I could care less about sex, is there something wrong with me?

If I don't "use" it, will I "lose" it?

If I have sex without having an orgasm, is that okay—or is there something wrong with me?

What if my partner thinks that because I don't crave sex, I don't desire or love him anymore?

My sex drive is on overdrive... I feel like having sex all the time. What message is that sending to my "conservative" partner?

How long can I get away with "later" excuses before he starts to look elsewhere?

If I'm not physically intimate with my partner, is this unhealthy for me?

Men ask:

What can I do to make my sexual partner desire me more?

How can I get her to initiate?

Why do women take so long to get "in the mood"?

My partner's desire for sex runs between hot and cold. What does this mean?

My wife and I love one another and have a good relationship, but she wants sex less and less. What happened to my once "steamy" wife?

Since she wants little to no sex, does this mean she's having an affair?

My wife doesn't feel comfortable talking during sex. How do I know if
I'm actually pleasing her?

As you can see, these concerns about sexual desire can impose stress on
a couple's relationship. Of course, I do get questions from women worry-
ing that the men in their lives—or they themselves—are "oversexed," but
the biggest concern for women is the virtual roller coaster of fluctuating
sexual desire. Most worry that if they don't respond to their partner's sexual needs, he may turn elsewhere for sexual satisfaction. And, of course,
they aren't solely worried about their sexual partner; they're anxious to
find a way to recapture their sex drive for their *own* enjoyment and well
being as well.

Why Sex Drives Differ
between Men and Women

The male and female brain triggers sexual desire differently. Women
have a much more complicated, finely tuned system governing sexual
desire and performance. They tend to have sex less for physical gratifica-
tion than to achieve intimacy or further closeness in their relationship. If
this desire to connect is not activated, the sexual chain reaction will not
be jump-started. To make this more understandable, I like to describe
this difference to my patients in terms of a light switch and a complex
control panel. In general, a man can become aroused at just the sight
of a woman; his response is triggered like the flip of a light switch. It's
a physical response. But women need all of their control panel buttons
to be aligned—all gray scales finely tuned and calipers adjusted—to get
them to even begin considering sex. By and large, if one little circuit is
out of alignment, a woman's desire is gone, or is at least greatly diminished.

According to Alan Altman, M.D., female sexual response is the result of the complex interplay among four major components: biology,
psychology, sociocultural influences, and interpersonal relationships.[1]
Thus, medication may not work for a woman experiencing decreased

libido because of relationship problems. Likewise, counseling may not be effective for a woman when a biological condition is causing a drop in desire. You can see the importance of accurately diagnosing the cause of diminished libido. And treatment of this issue may be complex (more about this in Chapter 7).

As researchers have continued studying female health, they are beginning to recognize that one size does not fit all when it comes to sexual desire. According to Dr. Rosemary Basson, for women, the urge to become sexual doesn't come before feeling aroused, but actually follows it.[2] That is, arousal comes first, followed by desire to become sexually intimate. This is generally the opposite of the sequence for men. Many women may find themselves rarely (or never) fantasizing about sex or feeling a sexual urge, yet when they allow themselves to become intimate with their partners, they state that they find sexual stimulation pleasurable and become aroused. Once aroused, they have more desire to continue. This stimulation can come in many different forms, either through physical contact or through an emotional stimulus, such as an honest heart-to-heart conversation.

How Often Do We Think about Sex?

Eighty-five percent of men ages 20 to 30 have thoughts about sex every 52 seconds! Women of the same age think about sex about once a day, except at the time of ovulation, the most fertile time, when women think about sex three to four times per day.

In general, the sexual response cycle of women does not follow a linear progression of step-wise phases. Women describe overlapping phases of sexual response in various steps that blend the responses of both mind and body. The strong correlation seen in men between subjective arousal and genital swelling/blood flow leading to erection is not seen in women. Rather, sexual arousal in women is strongly controlled by thoughts and emotions triggered by the state of sexual excitement. These thoughts, however, can also lead to more disruption, less ability to focus, and potential loss of desire to continue or be emotionally or physically engaged in the sexual experience. The following model reflects the state of desire for the majority of women:

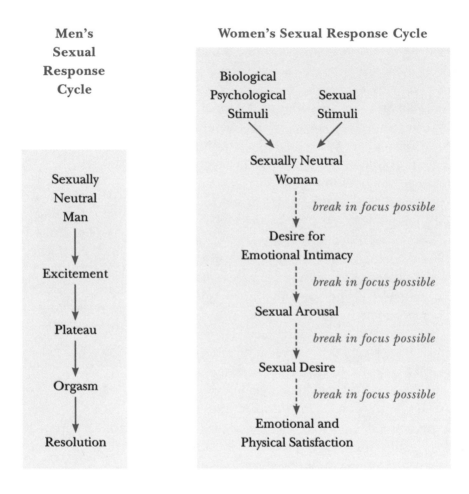

Men's Sexual Response Cycle

Sexually Neutral Man

↓

Excitement

↓

Plateau

↓

Orgasm

↓

Resolution

Women's Sexual Response Cycle

Biological Psychological Stimuli   Sexual Stimuli

Sexually Neutral Woman

break in focus possible

Desire for Emotional Intimacy

break in focus possible

Sexual Arousal

break in focus possible

Sexual Desire

break in focus possible

Emotional and Physical Satisfaction

The chart illustrates two important points: First, a woman's sexual satisfaction requires several stages of arousal—certainly more than does a man's. Second, a woman is easily distracted during sex! The message is clear: *She* needs to *allow herself* to focus and *he* will fare better if he understands that it is natural for her to be easily distracted. The problem is not him or his performance, nor is it her inability to be sexual.

Turning On the Light Switch of Desire When the Body Has Declared a Blackout

Generally, women are sexually neutral—they need a stimulus to make them want to engage in sex or become interested in pursuing it. The stimulus may be as simple as his holding her hand while they are walking or as complex as a man being an attentive listener. It may be giving her a soothing massage or running a hot bubble bath. For some women, it might even be a candlelit dinner that includes her favorite aphrodisiacs!

Women's sexual desire is more easily interrupted than is a man's. Several factors can interfere with her arousal, including the following complaints/questions that I hear every day from women:

- I feel out of shape and self-conscious having someone look closely at my body.

- I'm just too exhausted at the end of the day for sex.

- My partner goes straight for sex; I'd like a little more "warm-up"— things that get me in the mood.

- I just don't enjoy sex anymore.

- My partner seems "oversexed." On top of that, he went to his doctor and got Viagra. I don't feel I need to compete with that! How do I to keep up? What if I don't want to keep up?

- I'm often upset with my partner. Why should I reward him with sex?

- I've been on medication, which seems to be helping my condition, but it's killed my sex drive! What do you suggest?

- I want to please my husband, but it embarrasses me when he wants to try something new in bed. The more he tries to spice things up, the more I pull back. What can I do?

Frequently Asked Question...

What is orgasm and what is its purpose?

Orgasm, or as women like to call it, "the 'O' word," is a "climax," a literal explosion within both a man and a woman's body. From an evolutionary standpoint, sex is not meant to be just fun, but also to benefit in reproduction. In men, orgasm leads to release of seminal fluid containing millions of sperm whose sole mission is to find an egg and fertilize it. For women, orgasm leads to muscular contractions in her vagina and uterus, creating a type of vacuum effect. Since only 65 percent of semen is retained in the reproductive tract, a woman's orgasm with this suction effect gives an extra boost to sperm, facilitating their ascent through her cervix and into her uterus, ultimately meeting the egg in the fallopian tube. From a more emotional standpoint, orgasm equates to pleasure and a release of sexual tension. Sexual tension builds up in women just as it does in men. For some women, a repeated lack of sexual release can lead to irritability, frustration, fatigue, and a general sense of just "not feeling right." For a woman, having intimate relations with her partner, whether it leads to orgasm or not, strengthens the bond with her loved one and establishes a deeper connection.

Although achieving orgasm is a key desire of sexual satisfaction, less than one-half of the world is experiencing it on a regular basis. Globally, it has been estimated that only 48 percent of men and women orgasm on a regular basis, with twice as many men (64 percent) as women stating they do so.

■ There was something really sexy about knowing my husband and I could conceive a child. Having sex now that I'm menopausal just seems less risqué. How can I get those frisky feelings back?

■ I was molested as a child. I try to put this aside, but these feelings still creep into my lovemaking.

■ I've got a briefcase in my hand, the PDA in another, and a baby on my hip. There's just too much to do—having sex is the last thing on my mind!

These women's remarks are characteristic of the top seven reasons for low libido in women:

1. 24/7 life: Sex becomes a low priority on an endless list of life's obligations
2. Hormonal fluctuations: monthly cycle, postpartum, perimenopause and menopause, decrease in estrogen
3. Relationship difficulties: anger, resentment at partner—withholding sex to control/power struggles
4. Fatigue and stress
5. Medications/medical conditions/poor health of partner
6. Poor body image or low self-esteem
7. Previous sexual abuse and/or molestation

The Ever-Changing Libido: Stages and Phases

Many factors affect whether your level of desire is steamy hot or shut-down cold. One of the primary factors in a woman's life involves the hormonal fluctuations associated with different stages. Let's now look more closely at how libido can be revved up or shut down during these specific times.

Puberty/Menarche (First Menstruation)

Do you remember when you first got your period? Can you recall the changes your body underwent during this hormonally tumultuous time? Breasts started budding and growing. Hair began to grow in your under-arms and genital area. And what about those mood swings? This is the time

---

Sexual Myths

Cultural expectations, some religious beliefs, and societal views ingrained into us as children can also impact libido, creating "sexual myths." These are a few:

"Good girls don't have sex."

"Good girls don't like sex."

"Sex should be for procreation, not enjoyment."

"A good wife should always satisfy the needs of her husband."

"Women should never appear too sexually knowledgeable or interested."

"When women say no, they really mean yes."

"Masturbation is bad. It will send you straight to hell."

---

known as puberty, a time when estrogen, progesterone, and testosterone levels begin changing every day of the month. During this time, a girl's brain becomes increasingly sensitive to stress, with the verbal, emotional, and sex circuits becoming more fired up. For adolescent boys, the major increase in testosterone leads to increased muscle mass, hair growth, deepening of the voice, and a powerful need to express their sexual needs.

As girls begin menstruating, their brains mature within the hypothalamus-pituitary area. These areas send signals to the ovaries to produce certain hormones, release an egg at ovulation, and make progesterone to support the lining of the uterus in the event of pregnancy. If pregnancy does not occur, the uterine lining is shed and the cycle repeats itself. During puberty, a girl's estrogen level increases 10- to 20-fold, whereas her testosterone level rises only approximately five-fold. In contrast, a boy's testosterone level increases 25-fold between the ages of nine and 15.

So, how does a woman's menstrual cycle impact her libido? (Day 1 is the first day of her period.)

A. Follicular Phase *(days 1–14):* During the first phase of the menstrual cycle, the follicular phase, tiny follicles are growing in the ovary. One will

Understanding Your Teenage Daughter

Wonder why your teenage daughter seems to be on an emotional roller coaster? From years surrounding adolescence until the time of menopause, estrogen and progesterone spikes create weekly changes in sensitivity to stress, especially in the hippocampus (memory center). Your previously charming, easygoing daughter has started to react more to relationship stresses, and "drama" is the name of the game. During the first 14 days of her menstrual cycle, estrogen levels increase, and she is more likely to be socially interested and relaxed with others. This increase in estrogen causes a woman's brain to be most verbally acute at ovulation—if she's taking an oral exam, this is the best time! During the next 14 days (the luteal phase), she is more likely to be irritable and to want to be left alone.

But why is she on the phone so much? This is your teenage daughter's way to find refuge, feel more connected with her friends, and bond. Oxytocin is increased as intimacy is achieved by social bonding. So, don't get too frustrated with your phone bill. You might try to achieve balance by having a reasonably priced cell phone plan, and set times when she can use the phone and when she cannot.

become the primary follicle and be released at mid-cycle. Associated with this follicle production is a large rise in estrogen and testosterone. Surges in estrogen and testosterone around day 13 lead the hypothalamus (the main control center of the brain) to stimulate the ovary to ovulate. For the woman, these elevated levels of estrogen and testosterone increases her sexual desire. She has thoughts about sex three to four times per day. Additionally, she notices that her verbal ability to express herself is more acute and her memory for details is heightened at this time.

B. Ovulation *(day 14):* The egg is released from the ovary into the fallopian tube. All systems are go—the egg slowly moves its way down the fallopian tube in search of ascending sperm. Oxytocin, the bonding hormone, reaches a high point, leading to a higher need for intimacy and closeness. Dopamine levels are also increased, stimulating the motivation and pleasure circuits of the woman's brain. Her desire for intimacy and social bonding and sense of pleasure and well-being are at their highest at mid-cycle. During this time, she may be the initiator of sex, so her mate may want to be mindful of this stage of her cycle.

C. Luteal Phase *(days 15–28)*: The ovary begins to produce large amounts of progesterone. A woman notices that she's becoming much less interested in sex. Her levels of estrogen and testosterone decline, and sexual desire is curbed. Breasts become more tender. If fertilization of the egg does not occur, a chemical signal is sent to the ovary to stop producing progesterone, and the uterine lining is shed (menstruation). Then the entire cycle repeats itself.

Fertilization Occurs: Pregnancy and the "Mommy Brain"

Throughout the nine months of pregnancy, a woman's brain is exposed to high levels of hormones produced by the placenta. During the first 12 weeks, progesterone levels rise, leading to breast tenderness, fatigue, increased difficulty concentrating, and increased hunger pangs. Nausea and morning sickness reach their most extreme states between weeks eight and nine. Sensitivity to smell increases, and certain foods, even her favorite ones, can seem repulsive to her. She feels nauseated throughout most of the day, especially in the morning.

By approximately the twelfth week of pregnancy, a woman finds her appetite improving and the level of nausea becoming more bearable. Eventually, she becomes ravenous, increasingly searching for food and water. The levels of progesterone circulating throughout her body are now 10 to 100 times their normal level, making her feel more sedated, almost as if she were taking tranquilizers. Other hormones, specifically, cortisol, the "stress hormone," are on the rise. By late pregnancy, cortisol levels have increased to a point where she is becoming extremely vigilant about her safety, nutrition, and surroundings. Previous critical tasks such as making schedules and organizing lists seem unimportant, and she is

Frequently Asked Question...

We're supposed to have eight glasses of water daily, eight hours of sleep, work out three or more times a week, and get three hugs a day. One of my girlfriends has sex every night, and another isn't having sex at all. My partner and I have sex about once a month. What is "typical"?

There is no such thing as "typical," and every woman's desire varies during certain times in her life, within different relationships, and within different cultures. According to the 2007/2008 Durex Global Sex Survey, couples in Greece have the most sex, approximately 164 times a year, with Brazil following closely with 145 times per year. The global average is 103. According to this survey of more than 26,000 respondents across 26 countries, Americans fare poorly in the bedroom and in the sexual well-being arena. On average, Americans have sex just 85 times a year, about once every 4.3 days, which again is below the global average of 103 times (once every 3.5 days). The only global residents having less sex than those in the United States are the residents of Nigeria (84 times), Hong Kong (82 times), and Japan (48 times).

easily distracted and forgetful. During the nine months of pregnancy, the desire for sex can be high or low, varying within each individual and even within each month. Some women experience increased surges of sexual desire throughout their entire pregnancy, while others find an overall decreased drive for sexual intimacy.

The "Daddy Brain" and Pregnancy

Does a man's brain change along with his partner's during the nine months of pregnancy? A very interesting phenomenon, known as Couvade syndrome, occurs in up to 65 percent of expectant fathers. The symptoms of Couvade syndrome mirror those of the pregnant mother, including morning sickness, weight gain, and abdominal swelling. Fa-

According to an AOL and Cookie poll[3] of more than 60,000 American fathers:

79% said they wanted sex more often
62% said they are the ones who initiate sex
60% view online pornography at least a few times a month
54% have thought about having an affair since becoming a father
40% said their partners reject their sexual advances at least once a week
32% have had affairs
25% said they have sex fewer than 12 times a year
51% said they have sex at least once a week

thers with this syndrome have higher levels of prolactin and steeper declines in testosterone levels during the mother's last four weeks of pregnancy and first three to four weeks following childbirth.

Scientists believe that pheromones, chemical signals that stimulate smell, are produced and released by the expectant mother during pregnancy. The release of pheromones is thought to produce chemical changes in her partner's brain, preparing him to be an attentive, nurturing father. Prolactin, the nurturing and lactation hormone, rises by 20 percent, and cortisol, the stress hormone, increases by 50 percent, sharpening his alertness and sensitivity to various environmental stimuli. Two to three weeks after the birth of the baby, a father's testosterone levels decrease by 33 percent and his estrogen levels increase. No, he won't start developing breasts and crying at commercials, but these hormonal changes will lead to stronger emotional bonding with his newborn and a temporary marked decrease in sex drive. Yet by the fourth week after the baby is born, these hormones have returned to their previous levels and his libido will be back in full force. Thus, the comment I always get at the six-week post-delivery checkup is "My husband wants to know when we can have sex." If a woman has healed from her delivery, in general, it is safe to have sex. However, remember that huge hormonal changes have occurred in her body, and she may experience more vaginal dryness and less lubrication. I always tell my postpartum patients that lubricants will most likely be needed to make sex more comfortable, especially if they are breastfeeding.

The birth of a child can have a dramatic effect on a relationship. Women are often uninterested in sex and men often feel neglected. Communication between partners during these trying times is critical. Marriage can be a challenge and a compromise, but neither partner knows the terms of the compromise unless they both are open about their feelings, needs, and desires. Express your feelings and frustrations to your partner—it may well save your marriage during this eventful time.

A Woman's Sexual Desire following Birth

After childbirth, dopamine and oxytocin surge within the mother's brain, creating an intense bonding with her newborn. Thoughts of judgment and negative emotions are replaced by feelings of pleasure, attachment, and exhilaration. It is as though she is literally in love again. This bonding is further increased if a mother breastfeeds. Through the newborn's suckling of her breast, even higher levels of oxytocin are released, allowing milk to flow. She may become so attuned to her newborn that other members of the family, specifically her partner, may feel ignored. She is emotionally and physically satisfied, and the need for sex evaporates. She is receiving the same satisfying hormonal changes from breastfeeding (dopamine and oxytocin surges) as she would experience with sexual activity and orgasm. No wonder she doesn't even think about sex at this time!

The days and weeks following childbirth can be extremely trying for a new mother. If she is breastfeeding or pumping her milk, her levels of prolactin are sky high to help in milk production. Feedings every three to four hours can lead to interrupted sleep and irritability. Following delivery, many women will experience some "blues." And 10 percent of new mothers will experience a much more severe form called postpartum depression. They tend to be more vulnerable to stress, and levels of cortisol are much higher, leading to hypervigilance over the baby, heightened startle reflex, and feeling exhausted but unable to sleep. Well-known predictors of postpartum depression include a history of previous depression, depression during pregnancy, lack of adequate emotional support, and high levels of stress in the home.

In a February 2009 poll by *Glamour*, men were asked if they would rather be five foot two with a very long penis or six foot three with a short penis. Sixty-eight percent of men chose the shorter height.[5]

I have diagnosed many women with postpartum depression. They feel guilty that they are not "happy," worry that they are "bad mothers," and feel overwhelmed with the responsibility for their child. Many feel so ashamed that they do not want to discuss their worries or symptoms with their doctor. Luckily, at my office and other OB/GYN offices, an excellent evaluation tool, known as the Post-Partum Risk Assessment,[4] helps us diagnose and treat these at-risk women.

Again, I cannot stress enough the importance of communicating with your partner. Sharing your concerns can not only alleviate stress, but can also strengthen the relationship during a time when many relationships are being tested after the birth of a child. Your partner is not a mind-reader and cannot help you if he doesn't know what you want and need.

Libido during Perimenopause

The two to eight years preceding menopause can wreak havoc on a woman's body and brain. Monthly fluctuations in estrogen and progesterone still occur, but menstrual cycles become less synchronous—no longer like "clockwork" every 28 days, as they previously were. Now the time between periods is getting shorter, with it coming every 26 or 27 days. There may even be some skipped cycles—months where you don't have periods, followed by a month of very heavy bleeding. Along with stocking up on mini-pads and tampons, this period of time is often associated with a decline in desire.

Sex at Menopause

For some women, the release from worry about pregnancy is a major turn-on for more sex. However, for the majority of women, the decrease in the ovarian production of estrogen and progesterone leads to far less interest and sexual desire. Physiological symptoms occur with this decrease in estrogen and relative increase in testosterone. These include:

1. Vaginal dryness, pain with intercourse
2. Night sweats/interrupted sleep
3. Hot flashes
4. Changes in concentration/verbal skills
5. Irritability
6. Mood swings
7. Facial hair growth, especially on the upper lip/chin
8. Less hair growth in other areas, such as the scalp and pubic area

Although ups and downs in your libido can be alarming and potentially threatening to your relationship, do not become fearful that you are somehow "abnormal." By understanding the differences in desire between men and women, isolating the causes of your own lagging libido, and utilizing my suggested techniques, you and your partner can work within these relatively binding constraints. You will be better able to tame these seemingly unruly factors and increase your sexual desire, ultimately creating a more satisfying relationship and sex life.

Open communication is one of the keys to maintaining a strong relationship through these times when a woman's sexual desire is less than strong. A woman must listen to her body in order to understand why she feels uninterested in sex and she must communicate these factors to her partner. When he is aware of the hormonal changes affecting her negative physical and emotional responses to his sexual advances, the tensions that so often emerge from these difficult encounters can be lightened.

Frequently Asked Question...

Do women ever hit a "sexual peak"?
In general, women hit a sexual peak between ages 20 and 35. However, I believe that this peak can be achieved at any age—the key is being comfortable and less inhibited in order to enjoy sexual intimacy with your partner. As we age, we still see the importance of sex, with many couples over 65 years still having sex more than once a week. When and how to reach your sexual peak is clearly up to you—so what's holding you back?

Natalie and her husband resumed their date nights. She charted her cycles so she knew when her libido was at its strongest, and they arranged their alone time to be during those times. They scheduled enough time so that neither Natalie nor Mark would feel pressured into performing. They enhanced the effects by eating foods proven to have aphrodisiac properties. They created a romantic atmosphere with candles and sensual scents. But more importantly, Natalie and her husband talked. She openly communicated to him the stresses in her daily life and about the children. She expressed her frustration about her lack of sexuality but also explained in clear terms the reasons for it. Mark, in turn, acknowledged her feelings and offered comfort and understanding. He reminded her why he loved her so much and encouraged her to initiate sex only when she was ready. Natalie felt secure, loved, respected, and appreciated: In short, turned on.

Questions for Reflection

1. Looking back at certain times of your life, when did you feel the most desire for sex? The least desire? Do these correspond to the times described in this chapter?

2. What is your baseline level of desire? Has it always been on the low end or the high end? Much variation exists among women with regard to their inherent level of desire. Be aware of where your baseline is.

3. Do any of the sexual myths listed in this chapter ring true to you? Are you still carrying some of these myths around today?

4. What types of stimuli would get you more aroused and interested in sex? Think of all five of your senses: touch, taste, smell, sight, and feel. Make a list and share them with your partner.

5. Are you happy with the present level of sexual intimacy in your relationship?

6. How often would you ideally like to have sex? What time of day?

7. How often would your partner want to have sex?

8. Have you discussed your needs openly with your partner?

Self-Esteem: How the Body You See in the Mirror Reflects Your Thoughts on Love, Sex, and Libido

*"Sex appeal is 50 percent what you've got
and 50 percent what people think you've got."*
—SOPHIA LOREN

A PATIENT OF MINE, Becky, age 55, told me that she'd attended a three-day conference where she met a "gorgeous" man, age 60. He was articulate, bright, and attractive—everything Becky had been looking for in a man her age. Two dinners, five phone calls, and a number of steamy "I can't wait to hold your beautiful body" emails later, panic struck Becky: The attraction between them was leading somewhere.

She was excited, but also nervous at the thought of getting involved. Smitten, Becky's new guy wasted no time in booking a flight to her city to spend time with her. "Oh, no!" Becky thought. "He says my body is beautiful because he hasn't seen it other than wrapped in a nice suit and in heels that flatter my legs. But unless I hire a personal trainer and get rid of fifteen pounds, I'm just not ready for him to take a closer look at my body!"

On the other hand, Daniella, another patient, has absolutely no hang-ups about her body, despite the fact that she has quite a few extra pounds on her short frame and would never be described as "stunning." But Daniella sees herself as a perfect goddess. She loves sex and believes that men find her sexy! And this attitude apparently makes her very attractive to men, because she professes to have no difficulty finding men who desire her.

So why does Becky—a very attractive woman by society's standards—panic at the thought of a sexual encounter, while Daniella—who's slightly overweight and looks her age—become excited at the prospect of having sex? The difference appears to be linked to these women's self-esteem and self-image. In fact, our perception of ourselves can have a huge impact on our feelings about intimacy, sex, desire, and love.

What Is Self-Esteem?

Self-esteem is the value you assign to your personhood, a composite picture of your self-value. It's a "total score"—your self-appointed price tag, so to speak—which affects how you react to things. It is the degree of confidence you have in yourself to assert your goals, needs, desires, and values, to believe in yourself, and to believe you have the right to be happy and deserve to be loved.

A healthy self-esteem is achieved by actively participating in your life in honest ways: You refuse to be in an adversarial relationship with yourself, opting instead to be your own best friend. You respect yourself and stand up for yourself. You take responsibility for the choices you make and for your behavior—the ways *you* decide to respond to the people and events in your life. You work toward those goals that are important to you. You have thought about your values, and your actions are consistent with those values. You actively work to change those things that aren't working well for you—and are willing to self-correct when you recognize you are off course. You want to live your life actively and fully, as opposed to being a bystander or victim. You have thought about what you want, about how you want to experience your life, and you have developed plans and intentions for achieving this.

Therefore, your actions reflect the reputation you hold of yourself: It's evidenced in your choice of words used, your vocal tone, your style of communicating, and the value you assign to others (as seen by your treatment of them). Since behavior is a result of your feelings of worth and value, it's a telltale sign of how you feel about yourself.

"When life doles out lemons, ask for sugar." — UNKNOWN

Luckily, we can change our self-esteem. We can grow and enhance it! We get to decide! Even if you've struggled with self-esteem issues all your life, it's never too late to reverse your negative thoughts. It's never too late to "retire" defeating self-talk in favor of positive self-talk that contributes to a positive and healthy sense of self.

And the positive effects of a healthy self-esteem on your sex life are numerous. You'll become confident enough to know what you want sexually, and you will use positive methods to get it. You'll be able to initiate an open and candid communication with your partner regarding what you really desire and need in a sexual experience. You'll *allow* yourself to enjoy sex and be as concerned about being sexually satisfied as you are concerned about satisfying your partner. And a healthy self-image will motivate you to love, cherish, and have mutual regard for your partner, increasing the likelihood that any sexual experience will be positive, even if you're simply cuddling in bed. And this elevated sexuality will be a total turn-on to your partner!

> *"Self-esteem is the reputation we hold with ourselves."*
> — BETTIE YOUNGS

Enabling a Healthy Self-Esteem

Self-esteem is empowering and can impact all areas of your life. The higher your self-esteem, then . . .

- the more psychological strength you have when coping with adversity.

- the greater zeal you bring to the experiences in your life.

- the better able you are to develop and sustain nourishing relationships.

- the better able you are to connect with others who enjoy their lives and are working to their potential. Individuals with low self-esteem tend to seek peers who also think poorly of themselves.

- the better able you are to feel satisfaction from your accomplishments.

- the better able you are to relate to others and respond positively to them. You strive to be useful, helpful, purposeful, and responsive in your relationships with friends, family, and your significant other.

- the better able you are to exercise compassion.

- the more secure, decisive, optimistic, and purposeful you are: you become "empowered."

- the better able you are to recognize your own worth and achievements without a constant need for approval. This does not mean that you don't need others, but rather that you are interdependent (versus dependent) with them.

- the more responsibility you take for your actions and the more accountable you are.

- the more willing you are to accept challenges, take risks, and extend your boundaries, because you have experienced previous successes.

> *"A woman's face is a canvas upon which,*
> *daily, she paints a portrait of her former self."*
> —PABLO PICASSO

"I Used to Be 'Hot'. . . . What's Happening to My Body?"

Some women suffer from issues of low self-esteem all their lives. Others find themselves losing sexual and personal confidence as they get older. In speaking with my patients who are in their 40s, 50s, and beyond, I've observed that the age-related bodily changes they are experiencing make them feel less in control of themselves and their sex lives. As women age, they experience a multitude of bodily changes, many of which are not the most sought after, such as an increase in abdominal fat, dry skin, reduced muscle tone, hot flashes, and fears of incontinence. These factors often cause them to feel extremely self-conscious during sex, leading in turn to diminished sexual desire. As illustrated in the story about Becky above, they become more self-conscious about baring their bodies and may avoid putting themselves in sexual situations where they'll have to reveal their bodies.

Becky isn't alone. One study surveyed women at various stages of life. Regardless of their age or reproductive status, women were more likely to consider themselves less attractive at their current age and more attractive when they were 10 years younger.[1] Nearly 21 percent of the respondents could not think of even one attractive physical feature and reported an overall dissatisfaction with their bodies. Specific areas that women cited as the most dissatisfactory included the stomach, hips, thighs, and legs—all parts of our bodies that gain weight and fatty deposits with age. It appears that we have a real self-esteem crisis! And from listening to women in my practice over the years, I know that the more a woman perceives herself as less attractive, the more likely she is to report a decline in sexual desire or activity.

"I have low self-esteem, but I express it the healthy way . . .
by eating a box of Double Stuf Oreos."
—CYNTHIA NIXON

The "Cosmo Effect" on Our Body Image

But aging isn't the only factor that can impact a woman's self-esteem. Another influence is the media, which often presents nearly impossible images of beauty. Just pick up an issue of *Vogue* or *Glamour*, and the pages are filled with pictures of beautiful, exceptionally thin models and celebrities strutting in the most recent fashion trends. Do you ever wonder how you could get your body to look like those sleek, finely toned, supple bodies of the models in magazines? Sadly, many of these photos, even of women who are already youthful and slender, are "touched up," shaving off inches from their arms, thighs, and other body regions and smoothing away any imperfections from their skin and face.

I once saw a TV program hosted by Joan Lunden where she showed the hours and hours of work done to retouch *one* photo of Cindy Crawford. They took inches off her thighs, smoothed over her face...apparently, *Cosmo* didn't think even Cindy Crawford was beautiful or thin enough without changing half her photo!

As we all know, viewing those pictures of extremely thin and stunningly beautiful female models in magazines exerts a powerfully negative influence on feelings about our bodies. That's why in my private OB/GYN practice in San Diego, any and all magazines that show unhealthy images of women, such as photos of horribly thin and waif-like models, and those in which women are provocatively posed, are removed from our waiting and examination rooms. Who wants to see these photos and articles right before getting undressed for an annual examination? On a typical *day*, Americans are exposed to more than 3,000 advertisements—as many as Americans 50 years ago viewed in a *year*! Newsstands are adorned with images of impossibly thin, young, and digitally airbrushed cover girls, exposing their body parts as if they were objects for others to visually consume. In an article in *Ms.* Magazine[2], Caroline Heldman notes, "A steady diet of exploitative, sexually provocative depictions of women feeds a poisonous trend in women's and girls' perceptions of their bodies, one that has recently been recognized by social scientists as self-objectification—the viewing of one's body as a sex object to be consumed by the male gaze. It is a state of double consciousness . . . a sense of always looking at one's self through the eyes of others." This media portrayal of women-as-sex-object further implies that women *must* be dependent on men—we must do what the ads prompt us to do in order to attract a man. We must be thin to the point of being nearly invisible, young (a bit difficult to achieve if you are a mature woman!), and powerless. As long as we are in that vulnerable place, constantly striving to reach an unattainable standard of perfection, we continue to buy the products—and *that* is the media's main objective. And women willingly oblige.

My point here is not that women should stop doing things and buying products that make them feel good and feel sexy, but that "sexy" should be completely subjective and not dependent on what photos in a magazine dictate. These messages, unfortunately, affect men's ideals of "sexy" also. We need an across-gender campaign to be accepting of infinite definitions for "beautiful" and "sexy" so that everyone, women and men alike, can appreciate and enjoy the unique beauty in each one of us in a far less confining and judgmental manner

"I haven't trusted polls since I read that 62 percent
of women had affairs during their lunch hour. I've never met
a woman in my life who would give up lunch for sex."
—ERMA BOMBECK

Six Ways Your Self-Esteem Can Undermine Your Enjoyment of Sex

In Chapter 1, I discussed the importance of sex to our overall health. And in this chapter I've been writing about the importance that a healthy self-image has on our sexual self. Women must be careful to not compartmentalize self-worth and sexuality. We may be working hard and having success in bolstering our self-esteem, but then our sexual selves can turn around and sabotage our achievements! So when does sexuality have a negative impact on the health of our sexual identity?

When we haven't learned to love ourselves. Instinctually, we may understand the potential benefits of sex, but we may be denying ourselves access to those benefits by considering ourselves unworthy of them. We may know that sex can bring us closeness and healing, joy and love, yet if we do not fully love and value ourselves, we have not learned how to fully love others. This contradiction denies us the full sexual experience with ourselves and our partners.

When we expect sex to meet all our needs. Instead of avoiding sex, some women with low self-esteem use it as "junk food." Like sugar, it may bring them a quick rush, but it doesn't last very long. And though sex may satisfy some of their psychological needs, when they engage in it for the wrong reasons, it usually leaves them vulnerable to an increasingly damaged sense of self. It becomes a vicious cycle of engaging in sex to meet certain needs and becoming more and more dissatisfied after every encounter fails to offer the love they really yearn for in a meaningful relationship.

When our self-worth is primarily relative to our sexual identity. If we don't know how to love and value ourselves for the innate qualities we possess, we can rely too heavily on the outer trappings of life. We may then use our sexuality for acceptance, love, and approval and, therefore become sex or success objects. We want others to view us as sexy and powerful, but don't really seek to have them love us for qualities beyond our "sexy" attributes. The media, pornography, and sex industries contribute heavily to this distortion. They feed the delusion that women need to be young and always ready and available for sex in order to be desired by men. When women, young and old, accept this fallacy, they limit the possibilities for more meaningful intimacy. Believing our self-worth is equal to our sex appeal can impact libido in a real relationship because when sex is only about physical attraction, it becomes nothing more than a superficial connection that is easily broken.

When we use sex to gain power. If we have been abused as children, if we have never known love, or if we have low self-esteem and believe others won't want to love us, we can feel insecure about our abilities to attract the love and sex we need. We might even resort to power ploys as a means to get sex, which we may confuse with love. Power is the ability to influence and control behavior in others. In a healthy sexual encounter, people feel changed for the better. In an unhealthy sexual encounter, people feel humiliated, or sadistically enjoy humiliating others during sexual activity. They may even force a partner into deviant sexual acts designed to degrade and control them. Or one partner may act in a sexually aggressive manner toward the other as a means of getting revenge for being sexually or psychologically wounded by that partner or in a previous sexual encounter. That exercise of power is almost always concealing a significant insecurity.

When we become addicted to sex as a way to get "high." Sex can be exciting, and adding a little spice to one's sex life can be a good thing. But too much of it exposes us to danger, such as contracting sexual diseases or getting involved in sexual experiences that will make us feel embarrassed, tear our families and marriages apart, or cause us public humiliation and shame. Likewise, even though variety may be stimulating, if we indulge in it too frequently, it can objectify people and block us from the deeper levels of sexual connection. It can also be a sign of sexual addiction, where sex becomes little more than a need to score a multitude of sexual conquests. Or it can simply turn sex into bodies rubbing up against bodies, which in essence is no different from using others in a masturbatory way.

When we use sex to gain our partner's love and approval. If we are really only seeking to be held, cherished, and cared for, but instead we give in to sex when that is not what we want and need, we compromise our self-respect, and we lose confidence in ourselves that we are able to control any situation we confront. Additionally, we build up a deep reservoir of resentment and pain that can seriously damage our ability to relate in a healthy sexual way or to desire sex at all over time. In particular, a person who has been sexually abused and has not learned to heal these wounds can override her/his true needs and engage in submissive sexual activities that damage the desire or ability to have a healthy and satisfying sex life.

Seven Ways to Improve Your
Self-Esteem—and Your Sex Life

So, you have decided you are ready to value *you*. You acknowledge that doing this will not only improve your well-being, but also the quality of the lives of those who love you. You further realize that a healthy self-esteem is essential to a healthy libido. But you don't know where to begin on your journey to a better you. Here are a few suggestions to help you:

Own yourself. Know yourself. Trust yourself. If you don't like the person staring back from the mirror, do something about it. There is no time like the present to get on better terms with *you*. If you feel you need to better understand yourself or need self-awareness training, seek help from a professional, whether it's a psychologist, therapist, personal trainer, or life coach.

Keep your body healthy and fit. A fit and healthy body is a bedroom-ready body. But don't do it just because, like Becky, you have the opportunity to reveal your body to a lover. Whether or not you and Mr. Gorgeous get together, make time to create a healthy and fit body for your own good so you can feel good about yourself.

Learn to be assertive. Women of all ages can learn to assert themselves, love their bodies, and facilitate the construction of a new paradigm defining standards of beauty and sexual appeal in much broader terms. Actress Jamie Lee Curtis and model Tyra Banks have been quite outspoken about this point, but their efforts do not go far enough. If women demonstrate that confidence, *joie de vivre*, and self-respect are the sexiest attributes a woman possesses, they can stop feeding the notion that only a certain type of woman is sexy. Both men and women and their relationships benefit from this updated view of beauty.

Know your boundaries and honor them. Don't be tempted to engage in to sexual activities that you don't desire or that make you feel uncomfortable. Don't be afraid or ashamed of not pleasing the other person by engaging in a sexual activity in which you don't really want to participate. Healthy sexuality is about mutuality; it is not about force. Any partner who loves you or simply enjoys your company during a sexual experience wants to please you, too. He will not want you to pretend pleasure when all you are experiencing is pain. By learning to communicate what you want and don't want sexually with a partner, you strengthen your intimate bond and enhance the likelihood that you will have more reward-ing sex together. And do not be afraid or ashamed to say "no" or "stop" during any stage of the encounter. A respectful partner will honor your request. Talk about the reason for your apprehension.

Respect the boundaries of others. Naturally, it is also important to re-spect the boundaries of others in a sexual experience. Only people with low self-esteem aggressively coerce their partners into sexual activities. Engaging in such acts causes resentment, pain, guilt, and even self-loathing. If your partner be-comes withdrawn, disconnected, sad, or angry after sex, that is a sign that you have crossed a boundary, even if you didn't mean to. Your partner may not communicate that he has felt violated, so be sure to openly communicate by asking your partner how he feels after sex.

Be curious and open minded. While you should never do anything sexually that makes you un-comfortable, at the same time, be open to small changes that can spice up your sex life. If your partner wants to try a new position or make love on the living room floor, give it a try. Let's face it: while love is essential to a happy life, and intimacy is wonderful and nourishing, sex can become, well, sometimes boring! Be willing to be playful and to try new things. Take time for romance, sharing, dancing, laughing, and finding ways to stimulate all five senses.

Websites: Shopping for Intimate Products

Eve's Garden
www.evesgarden.com

Good Vibrations
www.goodvibes.com

SpicyGear
www.spicygear.com

Cultivate a positive and optimistic outlook. See yourself as a sexual per-son, the way Daniella does. Learn to see the joy in life and in sex. Be happy and feel blessed for your health, your partner, and the wonders of the sexual experience. Do not dwell on insignificant body issues or on a spat you may have had with your partner two days ago. Love your body and communicate with your lover. Love and appreciate every moment of your wonderful life.

Frequently Asked Question...

Is there such a thing as "too much sex"?

Most men would say, "Absolutely not!" In my opinion, there can be "too much" sex, especially if sex is used for the wrong reasons. For instance, if sex is being used to gain power over another, or is coming from resentment or anger, these are not healthy ways to express sexual desire for a partner. If you and your partner are truly enjoying and are physically able to engage in sex two to three times per day, day in and day out, I think you rate amongst the highest 1 percent in the United States. In general, the amount of sexual intimacy you and your partner have should be completely dependent on what you want, and should not be compared to some national average or statistic. In the ideal world, without all of the stress, worries, and burdens of your life, how much sexual intimacy would you want? By acknowledging to yourself that you may not be completely satisfied with your state of sexual desire, and thus your quality of life, you will open the door and enter into an entirely new realm of improved self-esteem, effective communication, and healthy intimacy with your partner.

As you bring a healthier sense of self-esteem into your relationships, sex becomes more pleasurable and enriching. Partners in healthy sexual relationships offer the best of themselves to each other and receive their lover's affection fully and appreciatively. There is no guilt or pressure in sex between two people who are secure with themselves, their partners, and the relationship between them. Love yourself, and then you can fully give and receive love.

> *"I admit, I have a tremendous sex drive.*
> *My boyfriend lives 40 miles away."* —PHYLLIS DILLER

Becky, the 55-year-old patient who struggled with self-image, thought more about her budding relationship with Mr. Wonderful. Yes, he often told her that her body was hot, and she appreciated that flattery, but she also recalled their stimulating conversations, the interests they shared, and his intelligence and good humor. She realized that their relationship was not based—and should not be based—entirely on their sexual experiences. Sure, being physically attractive for her new partner was important, but Becky realized that it was the sum of her qualities that made her "sexy."

There was no way that Becky could tone her body before he arrived to ease her apprehension about being naked, but she decided to be confident about the direction this relationship was going. She cleaned her house, went to the hair salon, and bought a couple of new outfits that emphasized her curves in a good way. She also called a local hotel for a reservation for her guy so that she could control if and when any fondling was going to happen! She bought a couple of bottles of good wine and invested in some nice, soft light bulbs.

Now, Becky felt ready to take charge of her relationship—and her sex life.

Questions for Reflection

1. How would you rate your body image? What parts of your body do you tend to obsess about or view negatively? How could you view these differently?

2. Have you ever asked your partner how he feels about your body? You might be surprised to discover that he finds you amazingly attractive and doesn't even pay the slightest attention to the aspects that you find most disturbing.

3. What are your strong qualities? Your sense of humor? Your compassion? Your creativity? These qualities are very attractive. Recognize their strength, and feel "sexy" because of them.

4. Have you or your partner engaged in sexual activities that have been affected by the low self-esteem of one of you? What steps can you take in the way of communication or counseling to remedy this?

5. What makes you feel good in your own skin? Make a list.

6. In what ways can you improve your self-esteem and learn to enjoy some of the healthier, happier, and more pleasurable aspects of sex?

CHAPTER 4

His and Her Sex Drives: What Was God Thinking?

"Being a woman is a terribly difficult task,
since it consists principally in dealing with men."
—JOSEPH CONRAD

JANE, AGE 35, CAME to my office wanting to know whether her husband's behavior was normal. "We have sex several times a week," she said, "and, as far as I know, everything is great! So why does Frank ogle the waitress with the tight skirt at the restaurant? And why does he close down the computer screen when I walk in the room? I think he might be looking at porn on the Internet. I just don't understand it. We have a healthy sex life, so why is Frank so preoccupied with sex?"

Jane was worried that Frank's behavior was a result of something she was doing—or not doing—for him. Was he on the verge of an affair? Did he have a sex addiction? Was he going through a midlife crisis? While Jane's libido was about the same as always, Frank's desire for sex seemed to be increasing. Jane and Frank had a terrific marriage, and Jane wanted to keep it that way. So, what was going on in their bedroom? Or, more specifically, what was going on in their brains?

Over the years, I have become very familiar with this recurring theme of a woman's dwindling sex drive and her spouse's need and desire for more sex. My female patients have told me about how they try to avoid the discussion of sex, and subtly hint that they are not interested or in the mood. And they wonder why their husbands or sexual partners don't pick up on the cues and quit pressuring them for sex.

As was discussed in Chapter 2, many of the differences in sexual desire between men and women have a biological basis. This structural difference in our brains begin very early in life, as early as the eighth week

Evolutionary Reasons for Brain Differences

Professor David Geary, University of Missouri researcher in gender differences, believes certain differences in brain structure and function make sense from an evolutionary standpoint. Geary writes, "In ancient times, each sex had a precisely defined role that ensured the survival of the species. Cave men hunted. Cave women gathered food near the home and cared for the children. Brain areas may have been sharpened to enable each sex to carry out their jobs. In evolutionary terms, developing superior navigation skills may have enabled men to become better suited to the role of hunter, while the development by females of a preference for landmarks may have enabled them to fulfill the task of gathering food closer to home."[1]

Geary additionally claims, "The advantage of women regarding verbal skills also makes evolutionary sense. While men had the bodily strength to compete with other men, women used language to gain social advantage, such as argumentation and persuasion."

of gestation, when the hypothalamus—the vital regulatory center of the brain—begins to form. In the womb, the male brain is bathed in large concentrations of testosterone, which prevents the male's hypothalamus from developing a sensitivity to estrogen. Thus, when fully formed, the male brain devotes more brain space to sexual drive as compared to female brains. It is important to remember that differences in the brains between men and women manifest themselves in generalized tendencies, not in absolute terms of behavior. By acknowledging these differences and tendencies, men and women can better understand their distinct behaviors and ease tension in their relationships. Rather than becoming frustrated at your partner's seeming inability to express his emotions, it helps to remember that, as a female, your brain enables you to express and verbalize your feelings much more easily than he can. Your emotional center is much closer to your speech center. Examining the neurobiological reasons for this and other differences between men and women

Male/Female Brain Differences[2]

Brain Area	Function	Female	Male
Overall size		Smaller	Larger
Density of neurons		Higher	Lesser
Area devoted to sex drive	Libido/ sexual desire	Smaller	Larger
Hippocampus	Memory	Larger	Smaller
Amygdala	Fear, anger, aggression	Smaller	Larger
Pre-frontal cortex	Control of amygdala	Larger	Smaller
Hypothalamus	Regulatory center	More estrogen-sensitive	More estrogen-insensitive
Pituitary gland	Hormone release	Cyclical production	Direct, steady production
Corpus callosum	Bridge between hemispheres	Wider/thicker	Thinner
Cerebral cortex	Selective skills	Language/ hearing verbal acuity	motor, visual/ spatial acuity

Frequently Asked Question...

Why are men always thinking about sex?

Men tend to think about sex much more than woman do. On average, a healthy, vigorous man will have thoughts about sex approximately every one to two minutes, while a woman will have thoughts about sex once every couple of days (and more during certain days of her menstrual cycle). These differences have a definite biological basis, with the dominant sexual hormones, estrogen and testosterone, dictating play. Men have 10 to 100 times more testosterone than women, which causes them to be more aggressive, more focused on a single task, and more directed in their pursuit. This effect of testosterone on a man's brain occurs very early on in fetal development, when a male embryo is exposed to large concentrations of testosterone—this is why men have 2.5 times greater brain area devoted to sex than women. So, it is no wonder then that men, in general, think about sex much more than women do.

is the purpose of this chapter. Knowledge of these differences can help give you and your partner the language you need to discuss the sexual issues in your relationship and to seek compromises and resolution.

Depression and the Female Brain

I have seen many cases of depression among my female patients. Not surprisingly, this condition can have a major impact on their sex lives. The propensity for developing depression begins early in a woman's life. Before the hormonal fluctuations of puberty, boys and girls have the same risk of developing depression, but by age 15, girls are twice to three times as likely to suffer from its symptoms. Intriguing new research has shown that there are definitive differences in certain neurotransmitters, particularly serotonin, within a woman's brain compared to a male's that may account for this difference in emotional intensity.

Serotonin, the neurotransmitter commonly referred to as the "happiness hormone," appears to be less available in a woman's brain than in a man's. Using positron-emission tomography (PET) scanners, a research group led by associate professor Anna-Lena Nordstrom showed that women and men differ in terms of the number of binding sites for serotonin in certain parts of the brain. In addition, women were shown to have lower levels of the protein that transports serotonin back into the nerve cells that secrete it. This protein is the one that is blocked by the most common types of antidepressants, known as serotonin reuptake inhibitors (SSRIs). Thus, women have less ability to spontaneously take serotonin back into their nerve cells to produce more serotonin. Not only does this variation in serotonin processing help explain why women are more likely to become depressed than men, but it also may help explain why men and women respond differently to treatment with antidepressant drugs.

The group also showed that the serotonin system in healthy women differs from that in women with severe premenstrual mental symptoms, or premenstrual dysphoric disorder (PMDD). The results suggest that the serotonin system in women with PMDD do not respond as flexibly to the hormonal swings of the menstrual cycle as that in symptom-free women. Studies have also shown the levels of circulating serotonin in women with PMDD to be markedly lower than in women not suffering from PMS.

Moodiness, irritability, lethargy, and unexplained sadness should not be dismissed by your partner as simply your "cranky mood," nor should it be a signal that you love him less than you used to or that you don't have affectionate feelings for him. When you both understand that these moods are natural and most often tentative (see your physician if they do not subside), you can avoid arguments that stem from these very female-brain phenomena.

Frequently Asked Question...

Why can he get all revved up so quickly, while I need more "start time"?

Because our brains are wired differently. Women definitely need time for romance, tenderness, and gentle physical contact before diving into sex. This is because women's brains have more connectivity between the two halves, or hemispheres, and communication between the left and right sides. This brain feature allows women to multitask much better than men. But this ability to multitask also causes women to be far more distractible and less focused during sex, which can definitely get in the way of steaminess in the bedroom. So while he is getting all hot and aroused, you may be thinking of the dirty laundry, the kids' soccer schedule, or what's on sale at the market. For a woman to get "turned on," she often needs to "turn off" her brain and focus on the present sexual experience.

Multitasking also increases the level of stress-related hormones (such as cortisol and adrenaline) in your body, and wears down your system through biochemical friction, prematurely aging you. In the short term, the confusion, fatigue, and chaos resulting from multitasking merely hampers your ability to focus and analyze. In the long term, however, it may have detrimental effects on your health, killing your libido along the way. Women need to do less multitasking and focus more on one particular task at a time. This will help them to live longer, healthier lives, and increase their libido in the process.

The Female Brain: Why Women Are Better at Multitasking

Though women often complain to me that they are exhausted from juggling so many tasks, the fact is they are wired to do so. Whereas men tend to focus exclusively on the single task in front of them, women are equipped to manage several tasks at the same time. This ability to do many things at once allows us to manage our homes and our work, usually with great aptitude, but this same "gift" also allows us to become easily distracted. Unfortunately, distractions during sex can be a problem. But I digress! Let's look at some of the physiology behind this natural ability to multitask.

In simple terms, the two hemispheres in a woman's brain are more able than a man's to communicate with each other, accounting for her greater ability to multitask. In the female brain, in the absence of high levels of circulating testosterone, the female develops specialized receptor cells that are sensitive to estrogen in the bloodstream. The high concentrations of estrogen during fetal development cause greater connectivity between the two hemispheres, or sides, of the brain. This connecting bridge is called the corpus callosum. The wider bridge allows for higher connectivity between the left and right sides, allowing a woman to multitask much more easily than her male counterpart. She can be talking on the phone while stirring a pot on the stove with one hand and holding a baby in the other. This is why women seem to be able to juggle five or six things at once, whereas men need to be able to focus on only one specific topic at a time. This ability to cerebrally juggle can affect her focus, however, and sometimes compromise her attention on lovemaking. As long as you are both aware of this naturally occurring response, and you can openly communicate, those occasional distractions will become much less of an issue. For a further discussion of multitasking and stress, see Chapter 6.

Why Women Are Better at Expressing Their Feelings (and Men Are Better at Reading Maps)

The centers for language skills are laid down during embryonic development. In the female brain, due to the increased levels of estrogen, more nerve cells develop in the left side of the brain, allowing for earlier language development and verbal ability than in the male brain. By the time a girl reaches adolescence, she uses three times the amount of words, approximately 21,000 words a day, as compared to her male counterpart, who uses approximately 7,000 to 10,000 words a day. As I noted earlier, the male brain, in general, is designed to focus on one thing at a time. If too many details are put into a discussion, his eyes begin to glaze over, and you've lost his attention to the conversation.

Due to the feminization of the female brain, even within a few days of life changes can be seen between male and female newborns. Females make eye contact, and start eye tracking and noticing facial expressions, within the first few weeks of life. Later in life these female visual qualities are seen in a woman's increased ability to pick up on visual cues and sense her partner's feelings, whereas males develop a higher ability to visualize objects in three dimensions or read maps, labyrinths, and diagrams.

What Do Women Look for in a Long-Term Partner?[4]
1. Personality
2. Humor
3. Sensitivity
4. Brains
5. Good body

What Do Men Look for in a Long-Term Partner?
1. Personality
2. Good looks
3. Brains
4. Humor

As children, the differences in boys' and girls' brain structures become clearly evident and are responsible for certain behavior patterns. According to Simon Baron-Cohen, professor of developmental psychology and psychiatry at Cambridge University and author of *The Essential Difference: The Truth About the Male and Female Brain*, "males tend to show far more 'direct' aggression such as pushing, hitting and punching. Females tend to show more 'indirect' (or covert) aggression, like gossip and exclusion."[3]

Women generally have a wider corpus callosum, which allows for more intercommunication between the right and left hemispheres. The brain functions of women tend to be more finely distributed, while men have a more "asymmetrical" brain, with more specialized regions for specific skills. This explains the difference in rehabilitation between a man and a woman following a stroke to the left side of the brain, which controls speech. This event has been shown to be far more devastating in men than in women. Women are much better able to rehabilitate, having greater ability to perform tasks and speech using the other side of her brain. Men have more trouble following an injury to the left hemisphere, resulting in more profound speech loss.

When my patients complain that their partner will not talk about what he's feeling, I inform them that the problem isn't that he *won't* talk about the relationship, it's that he *can't*. If women can guide the conversation by defining the issues and by asking their partner questions about his feelings, many would-be arguments can become productive conversations.

"Sometimes I wonder if men and women really suit each other. Perhaps they should live next door and just visit now and then."
— KATHARINE HEPBURN

What Attracts Mars to Venus

My patients often tell me that they see men as visual creatures who are affected by visual stimuli much more than women are. That is why during an intense discussion with your partner, his eyes might wander over to the woman wearing the low-cut blouse at the next table. Like it or not, how we look physically does have a visual and emotional impact on our partner. Interestingly, it has been found that within the first four minutes of meeting a new person, we have formed 90 percent of our opinion about him or her, and we have assessed physical desirability within 10 seconds! For a man, sexual attraction occurs on a biological level—he focuses on how a woman displays attributes that show greater propensity to successfully pass on his genes to the next generation. At the biological level, a woman is assessing a man's ability to provide food and safety for her during the child-bearing years. A characteristic that attracts a man to a woman is an "athletic body shape," which indicates she is strong and fit, and therefore able to successfully bear his children, run from danger, and defend offspring, if necessary.

According to evolutionary biologist Robert Trivers, women choose their mates based on certain attributes such as tallness, broad shoulders, and athleticism because those choices are a "savvy investment strategy."[5] Human females have a limited number of eggs and invest more in bearing and raising children than males do. For women, it is essential that they be careful with their precious "jewels" and choose that mate who will be the best long-term partner, protect them and their offspring, and provide food, shelter, and needed resources.

Although these qualities may have been conducive to the lives of cave-men and women—and still hold true at the biological level—today's woman wants more than just physical attraction to her man. She also wants an *emotional* connection. She wants a man who can protect her, but also be able to listen to her and to support her in her goals and ambitions. It's a combination of two opposite requirements: hardness and softness. American culture has indeed been experiencing a paradigm shift in tra-ditional gender roles for nearly a century. As women become providers and men more and more often become caretakers and nurturers, certain criteria for choosing mates may change, but it will likely take more time than several decades—a split second in evolutionary terms—for these characteristics attracting men to women and women to men to change.

> *"A lot of guys think the larger a woman's breasts are,*
> *the less intelligent she is. I don't think it works like that.*
> *I think it's the opposite. I think the larger a*
> *woman's breasts are, the less intelligent the men become."*
> —ANITA WISE

Brain Differences—and Their Implications for Ways that Men and Women Relate to One Another

The following are some questions that baffle the sexes, followed by fa-miliar scenarios.

1. Why won't he ask for directions? Sara and Jim have been dating for the past six months and have decided to take a weekend trip together. Friday afternoon, they leave Los Angeles in Jim's red sportscar and drive to California's wine country. At a critical intersection, Sara believes that they should head east, while Jim is adamant that the correct route is west, which is the direction they take. After fidgeting in her seat for 45

Frequently Asked Question...

Why do men believe that "foreplay" lasts only a microsecond? Why does it take me so much longer to get "revved up"? Sex therapists have told me that foreplay means very different things to a man and a woman. For women, foreplay starts a good 24 hours before any thoughts of sexual intimacy enter their minds. For men, foreplay may mean two to three nanoseconds before sexual intercourse. Why is this so? Women have the ability to remember things in great and vivid detail, and they can retain much more than their male partners. This means that if they are harboring anger, resentment, or frustration toward their partner over a minute detail that occurred perhaps even 24 hours prior, it may take an entire day to get over this before even thinking about becoming hot and aroused.

According to a Durex 2007/2008 Global Sex Survey, Americans spend only 35 minutes on foreplay and sexual intercourse each session, although they spend nearly three hours every week grooming themselves. So, it seems, a change in our priorities is in order!

---

minutes, Sara, frustrated, asks Jim to stop at the nearest gas station to ask for directions. He, of course, adamantly refuses, stating that he knows exactly where he's going and he doesn't need directions from anyone. Sara foresees that the weekend will not be what she had been fantasizing about. What began as an intimate, romantic weekend that made her feel excited and eager has now filled her with anxiety and uncertainty. Why can't he just ask for help at the gas station? As the tension builds between them, their hopes for romance and intimacy begin to dwindle.

Multiple factors are at work in this scenario. If Jim were to ask for directions, he believes that this would reflect poorly on his manhood. A "real" man never needs help from anyone else. Jim believes that he can navigate adroitly, without assistance from anyone.

Frequently Asked Question...

My partner likes to watch porn while we are making love. I don't feel comfortable with this. What should I do?

Watching porn before, during, or after sex is becoming more and more common. My patients have shared with me how potentially destructive the use of Internet porn or other porn can be to their relationships. In general, if porn is being used in a way to increase connection between you and your partner, such as for foreplay or arousal, then this can be beneficial for your sexual relationship. Yet if your partner is focused on the video/TV/computer screen to the extent that he is not really "being" with you, then this can be destructive. He is merely "getting off," so to speak. This may very well be the reason why you do not feel comfortable with it. He is not paying attention to you, but rather is mesmerized by the one, two, or three other women on the screen behind you! I recommend that you discuss this tender topic with him during a time far separated from any inkling of sex. This way, you can have his full attention without distraction and be able to express how you feel. When you communicate how this is negatively affecting sexual intimacy with him, and ultimately your relationship, he will begin to listen and stop this habit.

Sara, on the other hand, doesn't want to compromise the romance that prompted their plans, so she sits and stews instead of speaking out. Why? Just as with the animal kingdom, we are born with the primitive instinct for survival. More than 10,000 years ago, this instinct drove us to procreate to ensure the survival of the species—to produce the healthiest, strongest babies as often as possible, and as effectively as possible. In this model, there is little element of enjoyment with sexual reproduction, but rather the driving force was the essential need to reproduce. For a man, there was the need to disseminate his seed among as many possible recipients as possible. For a woman, on the other hand, sex was more of a bartering tool. In other words, sex was traded for protection and food. If a woman displeased a man by not cooperating with him sexually, she risked exposing herself to the threat of wild animals or sub-jecting herself and her offspring to an insufficient food supply. To lose his approval would be essentially life-threatening. Thus, women learned not to voice their disapproval, which is why Sara sat in stony silence while Jim got more and more lost.

Solution: Realize that you and your partner have different spatial abilities and navigational skills. Men love spatial gadgetry, so let him buy a high-end GPS system that will always point him in the right direction. This way, he's in charge of the ship, feeling like a man, and you are assured of not getting lost.

> *"Men can read maps better than women. 'Cause only*
> *the male mind could conceive of one inch equaling a hundred miles."*
> —ROSEANNE BARR

2. Why can't she just relax? Michael has been waiting all week for some time alone with Julie. Now it's Friday night, and he's hoping that Julie is "in the mood." He has the setting prepared with her favorite candles, soft lighting, and soothing music. As he snuggles up to Julie, testosterone surges through his body. He is getting excited at the thought of touching Julie's naked body and being intimate with her. He's on a one-way train, a nonstop voyage to nirvana. But Julie seems so distracted. Why can't she just be in the moment? Sure, Julie's mind has registered that the candles smell very soothing and warm. She's starting to feel more relaxed and wants to be closer to Michael, but what about tomorrow's soccer game? Did she pack the lunches and order the snacks for the team? What about after the game? Julie just can't seem to focus on the moment at hand. Michael's mind is on sex; Julie's is on plans for tomorrow. What's up with that?

Have you experienced a similar scenario? Thinking of what needs to be done, how to get it all organized, keeping it all under control . . . during what should be a moment of intimacy? Multiple thoughts fill our brains, telling us that we need to do more. How can we be relaxing, reveling in this time, when there are so many things to still get done?

This is where multitasking can be a woman's worst enemy. During the many hours of the day and night, a woman is lining up tasks, organizing, and planning. Of course, the trait of being easily distracted doesn't help sexual desire in either sex. Think of the last time you went shopping. Yes, it was just to pick up some milk and orange juice, but along the way, you noticed that the peaches looked so ripe and delicious, and they were only $1.50 a pound. And what about those lean chicken breasts, also on sale? You surely couldn't pass up that amazing bargain. Now your cart is getting filled with items you never intended to buy. But what about the milk and orange juice you came to the market for?

Solution: To get turned on, you need to turn off your brain. Give it a well-deserved break. Allow it to do just one thing at a time, not 20 things. Focus on the scene and your partner. Mindfulness meditation is a very useful way to train your brain to do this. Using this method, thoughts can enter your mind but go right through without needing to be fixated on. Have your mind focus on something peaceful or loving while you are caressing your partner. Keep bringing your thoughts back to what is happening to you physically—how you like his touch, his cologne, what is turning you on at that moment. This may take some practice, but is definitely achievable!

3: Why can't he understand what I need? Erika has had a pounding headache all day. Although she told Tom she wasn't feeling well, he seems oblivious to her pain when he reaches for her in bed that night. "I really just need to sleep off this headache," she tells Tom, but he's reluctant to take "no" for an answer. "Aw, come on, a little sex will take your mind off your headache," he pleads. Erika's not in the mood for sex, but she's even less in the mood for an argument with Tom, so she gives in. Afterward, she seethes about Tom's lack of understanding for her needs. Why do his needs always come before hers?

———————

According to Baron-Cohen, "The female brain is predominantly hard-wired for empathy. The male brain is predominantly hard-wired for un-

Female Sex Drive	Male Sex Drive
More diffuse	More urgent
More distractible	Less distractible
More receptive	More goal-oriented
More motivated by wish for emotional intimacy	More focused on orgasm/physical release

derstanding and building systems." Women are programmed to identify another person's emotions and thoughts and to respond to them with an appropriate emotion. Men, on the other hand, are programmed to analyze, explore, and construct systems. Intuitively, they want to figure out how things work and extract the underlying rules that govern any particular system. This allows them to improve their ability to understand and predict the nature of events and objects around him, but not, unfortunately, understand why their wife doesn't want to have sex.

Women's brain wiring may compel them to ignore their own needs and place those of others first. If they actually do admit that they have needs, they render them at the bottom of the list or fulfill them only when the time seems more appropriate or convenient. While this prioritizing allows women to respond to certain situations rapidly and efficiently, it can also lead them to neglect their own needs and fail to set appropriate boundaries. Often, when it comes to sex, as shown in the above scenario with Erika, when a woman says "no," she feels guilty or anxious. Her instincts are telling her to please her partner, but emotionally or cerebrally, she may become resentful and angry. She feels forced into something she doesn't want to do. And resentment is a big libido-killer for women. When they don't feel they've established an emotional connection with their partner, their sexual desire takes a nosedive.

Solution: Communicate with your partner that you're not feeling like having wild sex, but that a little back massage or gentle touch from him could help you feel better. (Communication with your partner will be further discussed in Chapter 9.) This way, he knows that you actually do want to be close to him and doesn't feel rejected. Interestingly, when a woman is touched in a gentle, loving way by her partner, she actually becomes more "in the mood" and desirous of intimacy/sex. However, let your partner know that just because he is giving you a massage, it is not necessarily a precursor to sex. This will develop more trust between you and open the communication lines for more intimacy.

> *"I want a man who is kind and understanding.*
> *Is that too much to ask of a millionaire?"*
> —Zsa Zsa Gabor

4. Why is she so grouchy all the time? Judith is 53 years old and had her last menstrual period more than a year ago. She is noticing some mild hot flashes, interrupted sleep, and mood swings. Meanwhile, her husband, Thomas, 57, is becoming more mellow and less argumentative. In years past, Judith would never challenge Thomas in debate over any issues, especially political ones, but now she is finding that these issues are increasingly important to her and she wants to be heard. Judith is uncertain about what is happening to her behavior. She asks me at her visit, "Why do I seem to be arguing more with my husband?"

———————

At the time of menopause, a woman's ovaries cease to ovulate, or release an egg. She is no longer of reproductive potential and cannot conceive children. Due to this change in ovarian function, the body makes certain hormones, specifically estradiol, in much smaller quantities. Estradiol is the most potent form of estrogen in a woman's body. When the levels of estradiol plummet at the time of menopause (and fluctuate during the five to eight years before menopause known as "perimenopause"), certain symptoms arise. For some women, these symptoms are mild and easily tolerated. For others, hot flashes, mood swings, irritability, and poor sleep become intolerable. This may lead some women to pursue hormone therapy, whereas other women may not need it.

Whereas we may become moodier and more easily agitated as we age, men tend to become mellower. The levels of testosterone in aging men and women account for this switch. As we age, men's and women's brains actually, in this regard, become more alike. In men, testosterone levels decrease, which tends to make them calmer and less competitive and to display fewer risk-taking behaviors. Women, on the other hand, at the time of menopause experience a precipitous drop in estrogen levels, causing the ratio of testosterone/estrogen to increase: more testosterone relative to estrogen. This causes menopausal women to often be more confident, less aware of or concerned about what others may think of them, more internally driven, and more like their "younger" husbands. The relative increase in testosterone also predisposes menopausal women to increased facial hair growth, specifically on the chin and upper lip.

Why do women tend to accompany one another to the bathroom?

The "safety in numbers" stems from a primordial instinctual need for safety. Danger from predators was once constant. In the absence of a male protector, women needed to depend on themselves, banding together to appear as a stronger force. By banding together, a measure of safety in numbers was achieved.

Solution: I reviewed with Judith the changes occurring in her body due to menopause—the marked decrease in estrogen and relative increase in testosterone. These hormonal changes help explain her increased desire for stating her opinion and exploring new territories in discussion, as well as her physical, bodily changes. Her husband, Thomas, is also undergoing changes as he is aging, behaving more calmly and becoming more communicative, due to the decreased levels of testosterone. In essence, as we age, we become more like our partners. After discussing the options for treatment—hormone therapy, herbal remedies, and lifestyle changes—Judith decided to pursue more "natural" ways to treat her symptoms: trying to eat more soy products, decrease her caffeine and alcohol intake, and exercise four to five times a week. All of these will improve her mood and her natural production of endorphins. I also instruct Judith that if she starts to develop more intense symptoms, such as severe hot flashes, sleep disturbances, or mood

Tips for Your Partner to Make Him More Attractive to You

Of course, physical attraction is mutual. Though women are attracted to a man who takes care of his appearance, she is even more attracted to a man who makes her feel loved and respected. A man who does both? Sexy, indeed! Ladies, you might want to tear out this list and leave it in your husband's briefcase or on his pillow!

1. Learn to be a good communicator. Take a class at a local college on how to communicate, make friends, and influence others. Go to your local bookstore and find books on how women think and feel. (Or, better yet, just read this book!)

2. Consider seeing a personal counselor or therapist. This will open you to seeing things the way your partner is seeing them and get you in touch with parts of yourself not previously explored.

3. Have a sense of humor. Women love men who can make them laugh.

4. Show confidence. Women are attracted to men who are self-assured. But, remember, don't become too cocky. False bravado and a pushed-out chest are definite turn-offs for women.

5. Have set goals. Women are attracted to men who are moving forward, showing that they are independent and excellent providers/protectors.

6. Learn how to cook. This stimulates the primal part of a woman's brain. She will love that you can literally "cook and take care of" her.

7. Learn how to dance. Women love men who can move on the dance floor. Even better, take a dance class with your partner. This will bring you closer together, both emotionally and physically.

8. Take care of your body, inside and out! Start an exercise routine you can stick with and get yourself in better shape.

Top Five Household Aphrodisiacs
(obtained from a survey of my patients)

1. He runs a bubble bath and puts the kids to bed.

2. He makes dinner (tasty or not, it doesn't matter—it's the effort that counts), and he does the dishes!

3. He plans a romantic weekend (sans children) at a spa resort.

4. He picks up his dirty laundry, vacuums the carpets, and shows a real interest in keeping the house clean—because this is how I like it.

5. Every day, he makes a point of telling me how much he appreciates me.

swings, she should come back to the office for a consultation regarding possible hormone therapy.

> *"Male menopause is a lot more fun than female menopause. With female menopause you gain weight and get hot flashes. Male menopause—you get to date young girls and drive motorcycles."*
> —RITA RUDNER

> *"Boys will be boys, and so will a lot of middle-aged men."*
> —FRANK McKINNEY "KIN" HUBBARD

Jane and I had a long talk about the differences between her brain and her husband's—and how that influenced their thoughts about sex. I assured her that it was natural for Frank, at his age, to still be preoccupied with sex, even though he was getting plenty at home. And I encouraged her to communicate her feelings to Frank so they could have an open and honest discussion about sex. At her next appointment, Jane assured me that she felt so much better. After speaking with Frank, she felt confident that he was very happy with their sex life, and that his wandering eye was not a reflection on her attractiveness or availability for sex. "I can't say that it makes me happy when he checks out the waitress," said Jane, "but at least now I know it's a 'guy thing' and Frank is as faithful as he always was. I can't change his brain, but understanding how it works has made our relationship so much better."

Questions for Reflection

1. Do you get frustrated with your partner because he cannot multitask like you?

2. What skills do you admire in your partner? Make a list and review these when you start feeling angry or resentful of him.

3. What specific things could your partner do to get you more "in the mood"? Write down 10 things that would get you thinking more about sexual intimacy with your partner and share them with him.

4. How could you convey better to your partner when you're in the mood and when you're not? Is there a certain signal you can give him to let him know that sex is likely?

5. Do you find your mind on your "to-do" list when your head hits the pillow? How can you sweep away these distractions from your mind?

6. Communicate your specific needs with your partner. For instance, how much display of physical affection do you feel comfortable with? In public? In private?

CHAPTER 5

Fueling Desire: Aphrodisiacs and Scents that Charge Libido

"Anyone who believes that the way to a man's heart is through his stomach flunked geography."
—ROBERT BYRNE

DEBBIE AND HER HUSBAND, Ron, needed a getaway, a chance to reconnect with each other as a couple, far from the hectic pace of their lives. So they arranged a date night that included dining at one of their favorite restaurants, with a nice fireplace and an ambiance they both enjoyed. After glancing at the menu, Ron reached for Debbie's hand, squeezed it, and in an enticing voice, asked, "Feel like oysters tonight, honey?"

"Trying to get me in the mood?" Debbie teased. As she reflected on their opportunity to be together, she replied seductively, "Okay. Oysters are my favorite aphrodisiac, too! Let's order some."

Aphrodisiacs: Fact or Fiction?

It's a common notion that oysters will help get your sexual juices flowing. But do oysters and other aphrodisiacs—foods that are thought to increase sexual desire—really work? Is it true that the properties and smell of certain foods can put you "in the mood"?

The word *aphrodisiac* derives from the name of the Greek goddess of love, Aphrodite. For centuries, people have been searching for magical foods that will stimulate sexual desire and enhance performance. Some aphrodisiacs have gained their reputation from their shape or appearance, such as avocados and oysters. Others are mixed together to create love potions, such as those that have been derived from various animal parts. One recipe includes rams' testicles combined with honey and ground-up rhinoceros horn! Other animal-based aphrodisiacs gain their reputation from the apparent virility of the animal source, such as the tiger penis. Turtle eggs, eaten raw with lime juice and salt, are also claimed to be strong aphrodisiacs. Sadly, tigers, rhinoceroses, and many turtles are now becoming extinct precisely because people use them for their purported aphrodisiac qualities.

Just because an animal has a reputation for being virile or sports a phallic-looking horn certainly doesn't support the claims that eating it will enhance your sexual prowess. So, are all aphrodisiacs a hoax? Or is it possible that valid medical science actually supports the theory that certain foods or chemicals can increase sexual desire? And, if so, how do they work?

There are legitimate aphrodisiacs that work by interacting with our own hormonal processes. As we now know, the main operating hormone in women is estrogen, and in men, testosterone, although other hormones, including progesterone, thyroid, and DHEA, are also involved. The unique interaction and balance among these hormones can unlock one of the keys to understanding sexual desire. Given the correct balance of hormones, sexual stimuli pass to the pleasure center of the brain, or limbic system. The limbic system then sends signals to the nervous system and on to the pelvic region, causing blood vessels in the genital region to dilate. In men, the result of this blood vessel dilation is an erection. In women, female erectile tissues—such as the clitoris—are stimulated, resulting in increased lubrication of the vagina, an increased heart rate, breast/nipple erection, and greater blood flow to the vaginal area. Due to the simultaneous release of neurotransmitters from the brain, particularly norepinephrine and dopamine, messages of pleasure and arousal are emitted throughout our bodies.

Are We Having Enough Sex?

According to the global study Durex World Sex Survey,[1] we are having sex:

103 times per year, or 1.98 times per week, or 0.28 times per day, or 0.012 times an hour, or 0.00019 times per minute!

Considering that sex is one of the most pleasurable, natural, and healthful activities we can engage in, these statistics seem a little low. Could it be that we aren't eating enough libido-boosting foods?

So, can any of these reactions be obtained by eating certain foods or even by smelling specific scents? The answer is both yes and no.

"Sex is one of the nine reasons for reincarnation . . .
The other eight are unimportant. "
—HENRY MILLER

Food Aphrodisiacs

While a romantic candlelit dinner with soft music won't hurt to get us in the mood, eating certain foods can indeed foster a desire for intimacy and play a major part in our sexuality. Research has shown that some of the best-known edible aphrodisiacs do in fact contain certain vitamins and minerals that contribute to a healthy reproductive system—and perhaps a healthy libido. Medical science can't guarantee that ingesting these foods will increase your desire—and certainly what works for one person may not work for another—but it could be a lot of fun for you and your partner to experiment with these tasty treats. Barring any food allergies, I highly recommend that your next romantic dinner include some of these items:

Almonds/nuts: A symbol of fertility throughout the ages, they are a prime source of essential fatty acids, providing building blocks for hormone production. The aroma of almonds is purported to arouse passion in women. For a special after-dinner treat, try serving almond paste, also known as marzipan, in the shape of suggestive fruits.

Asparagus: Asparagus contains high amounts of vitamin E, considered one of the sex hormone stimulants, as well as potassium. Vitamin E increases blood and oxygen flow to the genitals, and potassium is important for healthy sex hormone production. The suggestive shape of asparagus can help get you in the mood, too. To achieve the optimal aphrodisiac effect, I always recommend that you include this delicious, healthy vegetable in your diet whenever you can!

Avocado: Because of its shape, the ancient Aztecs named this fruit *ahua-catl*, or testicle. Virgin Aztec girls were forbidden from going outdoors during the harvest of avocados. Avocados contain high levels of folic acid, which helps to metabolize proteins, providing the body with more energy. They also contain vitamin B_6, which increases testosterone production, as well as potassium, which helps regulate a woman's thyroid gland.

Bananas: This popular fruit contains bromelain enzyme, believed to increase libido in men. It also contains high amounts of potassium and B vitamins including riboflavin, which increases the body's overall energy levels.

Carrots: Carrots are rich in vitamin A, a nutrient needed for sex hormone production. For men, vitamin A is vital for sperm production.

Celery: Celery contains a powerful substance known as androsterone, which is an odorless aphrodisiac found in male perspiration that has been shown to be a sexual stimulator in certain women.

Chilies: Capsaicin, the spicy substance that gives chili peppers their kick, as well as curries and other spicy foods prepared with them, stimulates nerve endings to release epinephrine, a chemical that causes increased heart rate and possibly triggers the release of endorphins, natural opiates released from our bodies that cause a pleasurable feeling and natural high.

Chocolate: If you've ever wondered why you receive an ornate box chock-full of utterly decadent chocolates on Valentine's Day, your partner may know more than you think. Chocolate has been shown to contain a stimulant, phenylethylamine, which induces a sense of well-being and excitement that is conducive to lovemaking. The natural caffeine in chocolate also provides an added boost by giving you more energy.

Foods that Cause Low Libido

Diets low in fat: A certain amount of fat is needed in your diet, as fats are the building blocks for hormones.

Hydrogenated oils and fats: While good fats are essential to pleasure, these fats interfere with them and a good sex life.

Excess sugar: Sugar overload causes blood sugar fluctuations that decrease energy, overall well-being, and sexual health. It may also compromise neurological and circulatory actions that are vital for healthy performance. These problems are often evidenced in diabetics. (See Chapter 7 on the link between diabetes and erectile dysfunction/heart disease.)

Crash diets: A sudden drop in daily calorie or nutrient intake may cause a decline in sex hormones and a lagging libido. Avoid starving your body of essential nutrients. Provide it with the foods it needs.

Eggs: Eggs have long been considered a symbol of fertility. In ancient Greece, the use of sparrow eggs as an aphrodisiac was prevalent, and the sparrow is also associated with Aphrodite. In India, the Kama Sutra lists sparrow eggs as a potency builder. In many Asian countries, fertilized eggs are thought to strengthen libido. Eggs are also a good source of cholesterol, a needed element in the production of sex hormones, including testosterone and estrogen. Recent research on eggs suggests that consuming them in moderation does not increase the risk of heart disease.

Figs: A halved fig is thought to resemble a female's vagina and is traditionally considered a sexual stimulant. Figs are very high in amino acids, which are critical to increasing libido and boosting sexual stamina. For a man to break open a fig and eat it in front of his lover was once considered a powerfully erotic act. In Italy, fresh Black Mission figs are served in a cool bowl of water and decadently eaten with the fingers to "set the mood."

Recipe for Love

Asparagus with Roasted Garlic and Pine Nut Sauce
Yield: 2 servings

1 head garlic
Salt and pepper to taste
2 tablespoons olive oil, divided
1 pound asparagus, trimmed and
   cleaned
3 tablespoons finely chopped
   pine nuts

Preheat the oven to 350 degrees F. Remove any excess layers of the papery skin around the head of the garlic and cut just enough off the top to expose the cloves. Place the head of garlic on a square of aluminum foil and season with salt and pepper. Drizzle 1 tablespoon of the olive oil over the top and wrap the head entirely in the foil. Bake the garlic for 40 minutes, or until it is golden and soft.

Meanwhile, steam the asparagus until it is tender but not soggy, about 1–2 minutes. Arrange asparagus on a plate.

To prepare the garlic and pine nut sauce, squeeze the roasted garlic cloves into a bowl. (They are easily removed with a knife.) Using a fork, mash the garlic together with the pine nuts and remaining olive oil.

To serve, spread mixture on individual asparagus stalks.

For additional Resources, see page 173.

Garlic: The "heat" in garlic is said to stir sexual desires. Garlic has been used for many centuries to boost immune functions and cure conditions from the common cold to heart ailments. Make sure you and your partner eat it together—and in moderation, to avoid the sometimes strong aroma effused from the skin after consumption.

Mangoes, peaches, and strawberries: All of these are high in vitamin C, important for making sex hormones and chemical neurotransmitters for the brain.

Oysters: Oysters have long been considered the food of love. As legend has it, the famous lover Casanova ate dozens of oysters a day, once even seducing a vestal virgin by sliding an oyster from his lips to hers. Oysters contain high amounts of zinc, a mineral used in the production of testosterone and sperm production. They also contain dopamine, a hormone known to increase libido.

Pumpkin: Recent neurological research has shown that the aroma of pumpkin pie is a sexual stimulant, increasing penile blood flow in men by 40 percent. (Unfortunately, this same response in blood flow is *not* seen in women.) Pumpkin seeds are one of the best vegan sources of zinc, which for men is crucial for potency and in preventing prostate problems. Zinc is also a critical factor in boosting the immune system in both men and women.

So, the next time you want to get you or your partner "in the mood," serve some of these foods to see whether they have an impact on your sexual desire. Even better, follow the recipe to the left as a prelude to a romantic evening! Or start your own list of great recipies and activities that rev you up.

It has been said many times that you are what you eat. Eating foods that support a healthy sexuality can make you feel healthier, more alive, sexier, more confident, and more beautiful. Likewise, sharing these foods with your significant other can elevate your relationship to a healthier, sexier level.

"Sex is an emotion in motion"—MAE WEST

"I blame my mother for my poor sex life.
All she told me was 'the man goes on top and the woman underneath.'
For three years, my husband and I slept in bunk beds."
—JOAN RIVERS

Aphrodisiacs in History

- Aphrodite, the Greek goddess of love, thought that sparrows were sacred, and therefore the ancient Greeks considered sparrows to be especially lustful. Because of this association, Europeans would eat sparrows, especially their brains, as aphrodisiacs.

- The ancient Roman physician Galen said that foods worked as aphrodisiacs if they were "windy," meaning they produced flatulence! Galen theorized that a "wind" inflated the penis, causing an erection, so any food that made one gassy could give a man an erection.

- For centuries, drinking alcohol has been known to provoke the desire. Of course, too much of a good thing can also have the opposite effect. A bit of alcohol can help do away with inhibitions, but overindulgence can adversely affect performance. As noted in Shakespeare's *Macbeth*, "It provokes the desire but it takes away the performance."

- Even the Bible includes references to aphrodisiacs. In Genesis 30:14–16, Leah and Rachel, two of Jacob's wives, go to the fields to collect mandrake root, believed to have aphrodisiac powers because of its somewhat humanlike shape.

- Many substances are believed to be aphrodisiacs because of the Doctrine of Similars, constructed by Paracelsus (1493–1541). He said that diseases could be cured by plants or materials that physically resembled the organ or condition being treated. That's why many animal horns (shaped like the penis) and even bananas were thought to treat sexual disorders and increase desire.

- Ancient cave drawings have shown hunters eating the testicles of animals they killed. It's believed that the men hoped to take on the characteristics of that animal, including its virility.

Pheromones: What Are They, and Do They Affect Libido?

Of course, foods aren't the only sexual stimulants that can create a romantic mood. My patients often ask me about the legitimacy of other aphrodisiacs, such as perfumes that contain pheromones to attract members of the opposite sex. Pheromones are airborne chemicals released into the environment by our bodies that affect the physiology and behavior of other members of our species. Recent studies have shown that human beings, like animals, produce, emit, and respond to these odorless substances.[2,3] Pheromones have been documented to influence sexual behavior in various animals, promoting attraction between male and female moths, snakes, monkeys, hamsters, and many other species. Pheromones are detected by a sensitive organ in the nasal cavity, which in turn induces the sexual behavior.

In a study recently reported in *Nature* magazine, Martha K. McClintock and Kathleen Stern of the Department of Psychology at the University of Chicago found evidence that humans also detect and are influenced by pheromones. Through their experiments in reproductive-age women, they found strong evidence that human pheromones affect physiology.[4] This may explain why some women who live or work together report that their menstrual cycles tend to synchronize.

A woman's physiology regarding her sexual response to a man's scent is complex. A recent study revealed that 400 women exposed to androstenone—a pungent pheromone derivative of testosterone found in male sweat—responded negatively or favorably depending on whether they had the gene OR7D4 in their system. Women with no copies of the gene reacted to male sweat as if it were a sweet perfume! Women with one copy of the gene were neutral in their response. And women with two copies reacted in a negative way and found the smell "sickening."

Despite the evidence that pheromones affect sexual desire, we still lack scientific proof that the use of commercial perfumes attracts the opposite sex through the use of pheromones. Of course, anything that makes you smell sexy certainly can't hurt! And if wearing a perfume makes a woman *feel* sexy, indeed she will *be* sexy.

Scent and Sexual Desire

Have you ever been cooking in the kitchen, only to have your partner come up behind you and give you a sexy pinch on the behind? Sure, you probably looked adorable as you stirred the brownie mix and licked your finger after dipping it in the batter, but it also might have something to do with the aroma of the food you were cooking!

Olfactory signals, whether naturally produced, like pheromones, or from substances in the environment, like your home cooking, can be powerful arousal stimulants. Humans can detect between 10,000 and 30,000 different odors. Women, in general, have a keener sense of smell than men. Thus, specific scents that induce an increase in sexual desire may be worth further exploration.

Recent studies conducted at the Smell and Taste Treatment Research Foundation in Chicago by Alan R. Hirsch, M.D., have shown that the smells of certain foods can be sexually arousing.[5] Dr. Hirsch, a neurologist, psychiatrist, and the neurological director of the foundation, became interested in the connection between odors and sex when he discovered that about 18 percent of patients who lose their sense of smell, a condition known as anosmia, develop sexual dysfunction. Could this inability to detect certain smells have some direct effect on sexual response? Can the smell of certain foods induce sexual arousal specific to both men and women?

In Hirsch's study of 30 women between the ages of 18 and 40, using vaginal blood flow as the indicator for sexual arousal, he found the preferred odor for women was licorice—specifically the candy Good & Plenty—which caused an increase in vaginal blood flow of 13 percent. The combination of licorice and cucumber also created this same increase in vaginal blood flow. The combination of lavender and pumpkin pie increased vaginal blood flow by 11 percent. The women also exhibited a negative response to several odors. These included cherry, which caused an 18 percent reduction in vaginal blood flow, and charcoal barbecue smoke, which caused a 14 percent reduction. Contrary to what the commercials would have you believe, male colognes also did not cause an increase in response, but rather were shown to cause a 1 percent decrease in arousal response!

Women's "Favorite Smells"

Dr. Hirsch and fellow researchers at the Smell and Taste Treatment Research Foundation have conducted trials to gauge women's sexual response to certain scents. By measuring the blood flow to the vagina, various odors were tested to evaluate arousal seen in the female study patients. Interestingly, the degree of arousal seen in women in response to scents was far less dramatic than that seen in men. Furthermore, certain odors actually diminished female arousal.

Scent	% increase in vaginal bloodflow
Good & Plenty candy/cucumber combination	13%
Baby powder scent	13%
Good & Plenty candy/banana nut combination	12%
Pumpkin pie/lavender combination	11%
Baby powder/chocolate combination	4%
Certain women's perfumes	1%

Scent:	% decrease in vaginal bloodflow
Cherries	18%
Barbecue-smoked charcoal	14%
Certain men's colognes	1%

To spice things up, remember to keep a bowl of Good & Plenty candy next to your bedside and leave the barbecuing to your partner!

Men's "Favorite Smells"

Dr. Hirsch also recruited 31 male participants between the ages of 18 and 64, and used 30 scents and 46 test odors to evaluate their response. The indicator used to evaluate sexual arousal in men was penile blood flow. Results showed that the greatest measurable increase in penile blood flow (40 percent) occurred with the combination of lavender and pumpkin pie scents.

Table: Increase in Penile Blood Flow Produced by Top 10 Odors in 31 Male Volunteers

Scent	% increase in penile bloodflow
Pumpkin pie/lavender	40%
Doughnut (cinnamon)/black licorice	31.5%
Pumpkin pie/doughnut	20%
Orange	19.5%
Lavender/doughnut	18%
Black licorice/cola	13%
Black licorice	13%
Doughnut/cola	12.5%
Lily of the valley	11%
Buttered popcorn	9%

Cinnamon in combination with licorice and doughnuts rated second, with an increase in penile blood flow of 31.5 percent. Third was a combination of pumpkin pie and doughnuts, with an increase of 20 percent. The least favored odors (not shown) were cranberry and chocolate. Hirsch also found differences dependent on men's ages and characteristics. In general, older men preferred the smell of vanilla more than younger men. Men who stated that they were having the best sex lives tended to prefer a strawberry scent. Those who claimed to be having intercourse the most frequently liked lavender, Oriental spice, and cola. Interestingly, and in contrast to the women, men responded positively to every odor that was tested.

Why do men and women respond differently to various scents? There are many theories. Certain odors, foods, and scents may remind us of past experiences or events. Perhaps certain scents bring back happy memories, while others induce negative sensations, making us less receptive to sexual feelings. As we know from research conducted on male and

Tips for You and Your Partner

Experiment with scent. Find the scents that make you happy, bring back fond memories, and make you feel more amorous.

The following are some other ideas for making use of scent to spark your desire:

- Think about scents from your childhood or from places you love. Recreate them and assess their effect on you.

- Experiment with different fruit scents and tastes, such as a slice of strawberry or a piece of banana. What type of reaction does this induce from you or your partner?

- Try various essential oils, scented candles, or massage lotions in the bedroom.

- Cook with your partner. Cooking involves almost all of the senses. Think of these stimuli and how they can awaken your senses and arouse your desires: the sight of the rainbow of colors of a vegetable tray; the sensation of butter and flour in your hands when kneading a soft, pliable pastry dough; the aroma of sizzling garlic in a pan with olive oil; the taste and sensation of a piece of dark chocolate melting on your tongue. And, of course, if you murmur "sweet nothings" in your partner's ear while you're cooking, you'll activate the "hearing sense," too!

female brains, a woman's sexual response to scent differs from a man's. Just because a certain aroma has increased a woman's blood flow to the vaginal area doesn't necessarily mean she's primed for sex. And blood flow to the genitals isn't as predictable an indicator of sexual arousal for women as it is for men. As the studies show, women tend to respond less vigorously to fragrant stimuli as compared to men, although women are in general more *sensitive* to smell.

My older patients often ask me about nurturing their sexuality. For them, the use of scents and other aphrodisiacs are perhaps even more important than for younger men and women. As we grow older, our

Frequently Asked Question...

Is it okay to fantasize about someone else during sex to increase my sexual stimulation? Should I be concerned if I need to do this to get interested?
Sometimes, you or your partner may need to fantasize about someone else to become aroused and stimulated. More than four out of 10 Americans enjoy sexual fantasies and erotica to boost their libidos. As with most things in life, moderation is key. If you are fantasizing about someone else every time you are with your partner in an intimate way, then there is a problem. What needs to be explored is why you aren't fantasizing about your partner. Are you still attracted to him? His body? His scent? These factors and many others will be discussed in this book. By not addressing them, you are being dishonest with yourself and your partner regarding the true state of your relationship.

sense of smell decreases. Older men tend to have more trouble detecting faint smells as compared to their female cohorts. Hirsch recommends that if you are a woman and want to induce male sexual arousal, bake something with lots of cinnamon and pumpkin spice. If you're a man and want to induce the sexual arousal of a more mature woman, throw away your cologne, light some lavender-scented candles, and buy her a box of Good & Plenty candy!

———————

Debbie and Ron found themselves eating a bit hurriedly as they exchanged soft glances and affectionate conversation over their sumptuous oysters and warm buttered asparagus. But things heated up even more at home when Debbie lit some lavender- and pumpkin-scented candles, and brought out the strawberries and fondue pot. I'll leave you, dear reader, to imagine the rest of their evening!

Questions for Reflection

1. Does eating a certain food put you or your partner "in the mood"?

2. Can you think of creative ways to use food when you and your partner are engaged in foreplay?

3. What smells invoke a strong reaction in you, both positive and negative?

4. Do you find scented products like perfume or after-shave to be a turn on or a turn-off? What about your partner? Do you have a "signature scent" that drives your partner crazy?

5. Have you and your partner experimented with any aphrodisiacs? How well did they work?

6. How might you use scents creatively to arouse you and your partner?

CHAPTER 6

The Stress–Libido Connection: Is Stress Killing Your Libido?

*"The life of inner peace, being harmonious
and without stress, is the easiest type of existence."*
— NORMAN VINCENT PEALE

AS A 36-YEAR-OLD married mother of three children, ages five through 12, Michelle always led a busy life, but lately it seemed to be spiraling out of control. Michelle was working part-time as a marketing analyst, volunteering at her children's schools, and helping out on Sundays at her local church. Then her mother became severely ill, and Michelle needed to fly to the East Coast every two to three weeks to be with her. Her mom's illness, combined with all of her other family and work duties, were making her feel totally overwhelmed. On top of all this stress, her chaotic life was causing a real strain on her relationship with her husband, Tom.

Michelle used to characterize her relationship with Tom as "pretty good"—they could always talk about issues as they came up—but lately she felt as if they weren't even on the "same page." Worse, Michelle and Tom hadn't had sex in over a month and neither of them seemed to care.

When Tom did initiate sex, it was the last thing on Michelle's mind because she was so stressed out. All she could think about was everything she needed to accomplish and how nothing ever got done. She needed more time in the day! What Michelle really wanted was to go out with her girlfriends and vent her frustrations over a cup of coffee. Sex was definitely not on her mind. Why couldn't Tom understand that?

Libido's Stress Threshold

Michelle's story is typical of the way many women are feeling these days. A 2003 survey by the National Consumer's League illustrates that the majority of Americans are "stressed out." Of 1,000 adults evaluated in the study, 39 percent cited work as their major stressor, 30 percent cited family, 10 percent health issues, and 9 percent the economy. Interestingly, in this survey, women were more likely to report stress problems (84%) compared to men (76%). As we well know, women are more likely to verbalize their emotional situation and not feel as ashamed as their male counterparts in doing so. Overall, men tended to worry more about work (48%) than women did (32%). Family concerns were the primary source of worry for 37 percent of women as opposed to 21 percent of men.[1]

While everyday issues like child care and careers can be a significant source of stress, a sudden change in women's lives—such as having a baby, moving, or assuming care for a sick relative—can put them "over the edge." This "superstress" can lead to physical ailments, such as headaches, neck and back pain, stomach cramps, and hives, as well as emotional distress, such as irritability, sadness, depression, and loss of sexual desire. According to *Reader's Digest*, "43 percent of us suffer adverse health effects due to stress."[2] And the American Psychological Association (2005) claims that two-thirds of all doctor visits are for stress-related problems.[3] In my practice, because the majority of my patients are women, I find that the numbers are significantly higher: As many as 85 percent of my patients claim that they experience the types of stressors I cited earlier, and that this stress affects their mental and physical health as well as their relationships.

Multitasking: Good or Bad?

One of my patients recently commented that her women friends seemed much more stressed than did the men she knew. In fact, some statistics show that twice as many women take antidepressants/anti-anxiety medications as do men. So, why are women more stressed out than men? One reason may be that women are the "air traffic controllers" for their families—in a word, they're doing too much multitasking. They organize family events, take charge of the household duties, and arrange schedules for pick-up/after-school activities, among a multitude of other tasks.

This deluge of tasks confronting women on a daily basis can become extremely overwhelming and fatiguing. A woman must quickly learn to prioritize each task and then deal with each in a conscientious manner.

In Chapter 4, I wrote about how the physiology of the female brain allows her to multitask quite adroitly. Let's now look at the anthropological reasons we are able to do so. In the prehistoric age, it was important for women to be able to handle multiple tasks, such as foraging for berries while keeping a close eye on the children. But today, given the technological advances available, perhaps we've carried multitasking a bit too far. If we're making cell phone calls in the bathroom, checking the email on our Blackberry while walking down the street, and arranging play dates for the kids while driving to the market, we've lost our appreciation for "the moment." We're no longer enjoying life. And it doesn't take a genius to assess the effect of this chaos on our intimate relationships, which take time and focus to nurture.

Many women complain to me that they never have enough *time* for pleasurable activities—like having sex. Multitasking can be blamed for stealing precious time, and, according to researchers David Meyer, Ph.D., and Jeffrey Evans, Ph.D., at the University of Michigan and Joshua Rubinstein, Ph.D., of the Federal Aviation Administration, the more complex the task, the more time lost.[4] When people multitask, the prefrontal cortex and the parietal cortex are required to perform these "executive control" processes. These interrelated cognitive processes establish priorities among tasks and allocate the mind's resources to them.

Meyer, Evans, and Rubinstein studied patterns in the amount of time lost when people switched repeatedly between two tasks of varying complexity and familiarity. In four experiments, young adult subjects switched between different tasks, such as solving math problems and classifying geometric objects. The researchers then measured the subjects' speed of performance as a function of whether the successive tasks were familiar or unfamiliar, and whether the rules for performing them were simple or complex. The results showed that for all types of tasks, subjects lost time when they had to switch from one task to another, and time expenditure increased with the complexity of the tasks. For the woman who finds herself feeling like the subject of a study about the amount of stress one may endure before imploding, time management is critical. And managing one's time should not be one more task to add to the list of things to do. Here are a few tips for making more time in your busy day:

- Delegate! Give your children and your husband chores to do and errands to run.

- Set up online banking and automatic bill payments.

- Carpool for children's activities.

- Minimize! The less stuff you own, the less you need to clean and manage. Your life will also feel less cluttered.

A recent patient of mine illustrated the difference between the way a woman handles the pressure of multitasking and the way men handle it. She noticed that when her husband is involved with a task and she asks him a question, he says, "Can't you see that I'm busy?" and tells her to come back when he is finished with his task. But when he questions her in the midst of her managing her daily multiple tasks, they *both* just assume that she can be interrupted and juggle three (or more!) projects at one time. And if she fails at managing all her responsibilities, she feels the burden of blame and guilt. The patient's husband, on the other hand, when asked to take on several tasks, will get annoyed at *her* for even asking!

This case illustrates an essential point: Women *must* learn to assess their capabilities. It is not essential to say "yes" to every demand placed on them. It is not a failure to say no. Saying "no" is something not only women need to learn to do, but spouses and children also need to accept. Saying "no" gives spouses and children the opportunity to do for themselves those tasks they have relied on wives and mothers to do for them. They become more independent and appreciative, and women become less stressed.

Sex and the Saber-toothed Tiger: What Happens When We Are Stressed?

So, how exactly does all this multitasking affect women? We are all familiar with the "fight or flight" response, which is triggered by stress. Basically, our bodies react to stress by producing adrenaline, the "fight or flight" hormone. Following exposure to a perceived stressful event, we experience an adrenaline release, which causes an increase in heart rate, dilated pupils, and more shallow and rapid breathing. Blood is shunted from the digestive tract to more functional muscle groups, such as the arms and legs. Reflexes are sped up, and perception of pain decreases. Within an evolutionary context, all of these physiological reactions would allow us to deal more effectively with the stressful situation at hand, such as running away from a saber-toothed tiger.

But many times, we are under chronic (continuous) stress, not acute stress, such as in the one-time situation with the saber-toothed tiger. This chronic stress and continual release of adrenaline also leads to increased production of another important stress hormone, cortisol. Cortisol is produced by the adrenal gland and causes blood sugar to rise in the bloodstream, providing energy to the necessary muscle groups. Of course, the release of this hormone would be highly advantageous if one were in an encounter with a frightful animal, but recent research has shown that when cortisol is released on a continual basis, the effect can be detrimental to the body. And these responses certainly do little for the libido.

"Brain cells create ideas. Stress kills brain cells. Stress is not a good idea." —FREDERICK SAUNDERS

Why do we get a "gut" feeling about situations, especially when we are under lots of stress? Isn't it interesting that when we feel stressed, we can feel our stomachs literally churning? Or feel our hearts in our throats when we are losing control? Or feel flushed, paralyzed, and unable to act? Some enlightening research on the nervous system offers an explanation for these responses. According to Dr. Stephen Porges, our social behaviors and emotional disorders are biological, or hard-wired. In his theory, known as the polyvagal theory, one of our main cranial nerves in the brain, the vagus nerve, is responsible for many of our unique reactions to situations that we perceive as either safe or unsafe.[5] We don't necessarily control this part of the nervous system, known as the autonomic nervous system; rather, it causes us to do things automatically, such as digesting food. The vagus nerve exits the brain stem and branches out to many organs, including the gut and heart. The nerve pathways have fibers that originate in the brain stem and go to different areas of the body. Those neural pathways that go through the vagus nerve to the lower gut come from one area of the brain, while neural pathways that go to the heart and lungs come from another area.

So what does this information have to do with stress? Our bodies react spontaneously to certain situations and perceive them as safe or unsafe, leading to specific bodily responses. Remember the saber-toothed tiger? Seeing this threatening animal would induce major changes in your body, with increased heart rate, breathing rate, et cetera. This also would lead the vagus nerve to send messages or signals to your gut and your heart. In times of chronic stress, a person experiences many gastrointestinal disorders, such as gastric (stomach) ulcers and a condition known as irritable bowel syndrome. Using the tenets of polyvagal theory, the person in extreme stress should employ strategies for creating a sense of safety or security, such as retreating to a calm environment, playing a musical instrument, singing, speaking softly, or listening to music. Even better, if you're under stress, seek the safety and security of your lover's arms and talk openly about the troubles you are experiencing.

Enter Hormones

We've just seen what happens with adrenaline, the "fight or flight" hormone, and cortisol, the stress hormone, when women are under extreme stress. But how are the sex hormones—estrogen and progesterone—impacted by stress? Why does all this stress affect our love lives?

As discussed in Chapter 4, women have more white matter in the pre-

frontal cortex of the brain as compared to men. This area controls deci-
sion-making processes and regulates emotional responses to the world.
Messages from the prefrontal cortex are then sent to the hippocampus,
the main memory storage area of the brain. During times of stress, levels
of cortisol increase. Women—with their increased levels of estrogen—
will have increased activation of the neurons within the hippocampus.
This causes their brains to experience the stressful event more intensely
and vividly. A woman's recollection will be crystal-clear, with incredibly
intricate detail. Testosterone, on the other hand, found in greater abun-
dance in men, blocks the effects of cortisol, so the memory of a stressful
event is not as vivid or detailed and is not stored as efficiently. This helps
explain why women tend to perseverate on the most minute details of a
stressful event, whereas men tend not to be as affected. Hence, the well-
known phrase: "Men never remember, and women never forget!"

If you are a woman, think about a recent argument you had with your
partner. Can you remember most of the details of the argument? Did
you continue to analyze each statement made, going over each detail a
hundred times? Did your partner, however, seem to move on relatively
quickly? Your hormones can be blamed for some of these differences.

"Tend and Befriend"

In response to the varying effects of hormones, men and women respond
differently when exposed to stressful events. When you have experienced
stress—an argument with your boss, problems with your relationship, issues with your child's schoolwork—did you call a friend, your sister, or
your mom to chat about it? Well, this response was actually biological.
In a recent study, Laura Cousin Klein, Ph.D., and Shelley Taylor, Ph.D.,
discovered that when a woman is under stress, her oxytocin levels rise.[6]
And C. Sue Carter, Ph.D.,[7] co-director of the Brain Body Center of the
University of Illinois, has found that the effects of oxytocin are stronger
when we are undergoing stress.[7] This hormone—released from the pituitary gland, a small gland in the inferior aspect of the brain—causes
women to seek help in the form of bonding with other women, allowing

them to calm down from the stressful situation. In Klein and Taylor's study, women sought solace in caring for their children and turning to other women for support in times of stress. The researchers coined this phenomenon "tend and befriend." This response to stress leads women to seek more social interaction, verbal communication, and close friendships, as we saw in the example with Michelle.

For men, however, the response to stress is different. Testosterone, the predominant sex hormone in men, counteracts the effects of oxytocin. This phenomenon helps to explain why men tend *not* to seek out other male friends in times of stress, but rather are more likely to become angry, hostile, or withdrawn from others. Men don't like to admit there are relationship problems because that makes them feel as if they have failed, a situation they find very threatening. They're more likely to cope with stress by vegging out in front of the TV.

All these biological facts lead us to understand why women feel less amorous when they are under stress. Estrogen causes women to experience more stress, create more vivid memories of the stressful situation, and retain the memory longer. These relatively exaggerated responses to stress distract her from thoughts of sex and prevent her from relaxing enough to enjoy it. Men, on the other hand, tend to alleviate the stress of a situation sooner than do women. Following a heated argument, men are often able to divert their attention to a completely different topic rather than to dwell, as women tend to do, on a previous disagreement. Men may even consider the possibility of sex after an argument! Why not? From their perspective, the conversation may have been a bit contentious but nothing too destructive, and definitely something that a little sex could smooth out! Women, on the other hand, can't even imagine the thought of sex at such a time, much less think about being close to their partner, and wonder how he could consider it. These differences can cause a real strain in the relationship and negatively impact couples' sex lives. At the end of the chapter, I will suggest ways for women to negotiate the harmful consequences stress has on their sex lives.

How Much Stress Are You Under?

Now that you know the harmful effects of stress on your life and your libido, think about your own stress level. Ask yourself the following:

- Are you experiencing a lot of stress in your life right now?

- What are the causes of that stress?

- Have you noticed a corresponding lessening of sexual desire?

- Do you find it more difficult than your partner to "forgive and forget" after an argument?

- Does it infuriate you when your husband is ready for sex when you're still stewing about something?

- Are you willing to alter the factors in your life that are causing you stress?

The following is a simple test to assess your level of stress based on events in the previous year of your life. I adapted this test from the Holmes and Rahe stress test to make it more applicable to women, but you may take the more comprehensive version at www.stress-management.net/stress-test.htm.[8] For the following test, place a check mark in the box next to the events or issues that you have experienced in your life the past year. The more check marks, the more stress in your life. But keep in mind that even one check mark can significantly affect your stress levels and, ultimately, your sex life.

Quiz: How Stressed Out Are You?
_____ Death or illness of a close friend or family member
_____ Major personal illness or injury
_____ Work-related problems, such as job insecurity, changing jobs or

careers, a change in work duties, a promotion, trouble with the boss, change in work hours or conditions

_____ Financial problems, such as being fired or laid off, filing for bankruptcy, assuming a mortgage or experiencing foreclosure, or making a major purchase (house, car, etc.)

_____ Pregnancy

_____ Miscarriage or infertility difficulties

_____ Expanding your family through birth, adoption, or remarriage

_____ Major increase in fights with spouse

_____ Son or daughter leaving home

_____ In-law troubles

_____ Spouse and/or you retire

_____ Going back to school

_____ Moving, rebuilding, or remodeling

_____ Experiencing a natural disaster (hurricane, tornado, etc.)

_____ Major change in sleeping habits

_____ Major change in eating habits (going on a diet, etc.)

_____ Planning or taking a vacation

_____ Christmas or holiday observances

Please remember, the impact of these stressors is not absolute and can vary among individuals. Each of us copes with change and reacts to different life events in varying ways, and the availability of support through family, work, and friends is unique. These variables all impact how well (or poorly) we deal with stress.

> *"Over the years, your bodies become*
> *walking autobiographies, telling friends and strangers alike*
> *of the minor and major stresses of your lives."*
> —MARILYN FERGUSON

Reducing the Stress in Your Life

So, what's a woman to do? Short of running away to an island resort and leaving all of your problems behind, how can you get beyond the stress in your life and recapture your desire for sex? How can lifestyle changes help you to better manage stress? Below are some stress-reduction techniques that I have compiled from many resources, including some sage advice from my patients. Choose one or more of these techniques and see what fits you best. Keep in mind that what works for you may not necessarily work for your best friend or sister.

I recommend that all of the lifestyle habits be immediately implemented into your life. Make the decision to start today!

Common Techniques for Stress Relief

Diaphragmatic Breathing (Abdominal Breathing): Stress often causes our breathing to be shallow and this often frightening effect can cause more stress because it puts less oxygen in the bloodstream and increases muscle tension. The next time you feel stressed, take a minute to slow down and breathe deeply. Breathe in through your nose and out through your mouth, inhaling enough so that your lower abdomen rises and falls. Count slowly from 1 to 5 as you exhale.

Progressive Muscle Relaxation (PMR): Progressive muscle relaxation exercises release tension in certain muscle groups and allow you to then totally relax them. Some resources for PMR techniques are listed at the end of this chapter.

Meditation: Engage in exercises that enable you to focus on your breathing, on an object, or on your body's sensations. You want to relax your mind, body, and spirit. (See resources for meditation techniques at the end of this chapter.)

Yoga: Sign up for a yoga class or purchase a yoga video. Yoga helps you build up a natural response to stress and brings more relaxation into your daily life.

Tai Chi: Tai Chi teaches you to focus on your breath and on the beauty of the present moment.

Massage: A theraputic massage provides deep relaxation and improves physiological processes. Your entire body relaxes as your muscles relax, positively impacting your overstressed mind.

Craniosacral Therapy: Using refined skills of palpation, support, and light touch, a craniosacral therapist works with the cerebral fluid, fascia, tides in the body, the limbic system, and all factors related to stress and imbalance.

Acupuncture: Very fine needles the diameter of a cat's whisker are specifically placed on the skin to target certain points in order to alleviate pain, swelling, and stress.

Bodywork: Bodywork is therapy that involves some form of touching, energy work, or physical manipulation of the body.

Physical Therapy: Physical therapy is performed to help people develop, maintain, or restore movement and functioning.

Five Suggestions for Managing Stress— and Upping Your Libido

Nobody will ever have a stress-free life, but you can do plenty to minimize your anxiety and put the fun back into living—and your relationship! Try these suggestions:

1. Prioritize what's most important in your life: Make a list of all the stressful things in your life . . . everything! (The quiz you took in this chapter is a good place to start.) Then go through the list and evaluate which activities bring you enjoyment, which you have to do to survive, and which you may be doing solely out of obligation/guilt. Resolve to eliminate those things from your life that are stressing you out. If you feel resentful that you've been put in charge of the PTA bake sale for the

third year in a row, hand over the reins! Let someone else take a turn this year. Make lifestyle changes to become more organized and manage your time better, and consider deleting certain activities that you really don't enjoy. Do you need to get a family calendar to keep track of everyone's schedule? Can you put out the next day's clothes and breakfast dishes the night before to avoid early-morning stress? Once you've cleared your schedule a bit, add some time back in that allows you to do something for yourself every day. When we're always doing for others and neglecting ourselves, resentment can build up—a significant source of stress. Put yourself first by taking a walk, having a cup of tea with a friend, taking a warm bath, or scheduling a massage.

2. **Exercise:** Make time to exercise at least 30 minutes at a time, three to four times per week. Physical activity plays a key role in reducing and preventing the effects of stress. Forms of exercise could range from walking in the park/beach/neighborhood, going for a run/fast walk, or going to the gym (aerobics/spinning/weights, etc.). And it's just as important to "exercise" your mind through relaxing activities such as yoga, meditation, listening to music, petting your cat/dog, pursuing a hobby, or writing in a journal. Schedule these activities into your week, just as you would a doctor's appointment or work obligation. Give them high priority in your life. Invite your partner to join you! Shared enjoyable activities will bring you closer together.

3. **Improve your sleeping habits:** Some of us need only five to six hours of sleep per night, while others require a full eight or more hours. Giving yourself adequate sleep refuels your mind, as well as your body. If you always seem tired, take a good look at your sleeping habits. You may not be getting the quantity and/or quality of rest you need. Perhaps a sleep assessment or therapy is called for if you never seem to get a restful sleep.

4. **Connect with others:** As mentioned in this chapter, women seek out friends to bond with in times of stress. Develop a support system and share your feelings. Call a friend, family member, teacher, counselor, or clergy person who can help you see your problems in a different light.

Frequently Asked Question...

I have an all-encompassing job. How can I (quickly) shift from a more "bottom-line" world to feeling more soft and feminine when I get home?

Women who work in high-powered, male-dominated fields often feel like they are constantly swimming upstream to keep up with their male counterparts. They need to behave in a certain manner with men in the workplace to gain respect and be taken seriously. Unfortunately, these same behaviors, which are often masculine characteristics, can be destructive at home. I recommend to my patients that they set aside a certain amount of time—approximately 15 to 30 minutes—to decompress upon arriving home from the workplace. Men already do this—they take off their shoes, change their clothes, and read the paper in their lounge chair. Why don't women? Because we don't allow ourselves to. But we need to! We need to have a "decompression time"—time to unwind from the fury of the workplace, let all of the daily trials and tribulations go, and just breathe easily at home. During this time, I recommend that you change your clothes, take a shower or bath, read a magazine, meditate, or simply take some deep breaths. Taking off your shoes and changing your clothes is like peeling off the layers of work-related images. Change into a pair of soft, plush sweats and a comfortable top. Dab a little of your favorite perfume on your neck. Light some candles and put on some soft music. Try to make time to take a bath—or, even better, have your partner run a bubble bath for you. By doing just a few of these easy things, you will regain your feminine side, feel more like a "woman," and maybe even start thinking about getting closer to your partner. This is will be covered in more detail in chapter 9, "Heart to Heart: Using Communication to Resuscitate Your Libido."

5. Pay attention to what you put in your body: Your body is your palace—what you put into it reflects on you. Make sure to take time to eat breakfast in the morning. Eat five to six small, nutritious meals throughout the

Healthy Protein Snacks

- Hummus spread on whole-wheat crackers or a whole-wheat bagel

- A bowl of whole-grain cereal with milk and berries (Berries also add fiber and antioxidants.)

- Peanut butter on apple slices

- Homemade bran muffins made with milk and eggs

- Fruit smoothie made with plain, nonfat yogurt and fruits

- Celery dipped in low-fat cottage cheese

- Nonfat yogurt sprinkled with low-fat granola

- Edamame (You can find this soybean snack in the frozen foods section. Boil briefly in salted water—delicious!)

day, rather than three large meals. This allows for more stable glucose levels throughout your day, improving brain function and maintaining energy. Avoid consuming too much caffeine and sugar. Having two to three Diet Cokes or Starbucks coffees each day can cause you to feel temporary "highs" that then lead to fatigue or "crashes" later. Eat high-protein foods and recommended healthy snack foods. (See box above.) Foods containing tryptophan, such as turkey, dairy, and soy products, can have a calming effect, as can chamomile tea. Avoid self-medicating with drugs or alcohol. One alcoholic drink per day is currently recommended for women to prevent heart disease, but two or more is not. Although drinking alcohol may initially appear to alleviate stress, it is only temporary. Do not mask the issue at hand. If you find that you are increasingly turning to "the bottle" to deal with stress, seek guidance from a therapist or counselor to deal with your stressful issues and confront them head-on.

By using techniques to lessen the amount of stress in your life—especially those situations that cause tension between you and your partner—you can put yourself back on the road to a more satisfying sex life.

"Smooth seas do not make skillful sailors."—AFRICAN PROVERB

Can Stress Ever Be Good for You?

All this information about the negative effects of stress may just add to our reasons to worry. But because our bodies and brains are so well-equipped to handle it, many researchers have been wondering how we might use stress to our advantage. According to the *Newsweek* article "Who Says Stress Is Bad for You?"9, *some* stress can actually be beneficial. Because of the release of adrenaline and cortisol, it in fact sharpens memory and reflexes. Furthermore, exposure to stress creates a protective "memory." The same article cites a study conducted by Salvatore Maddi, a psychologist at the University of California, Irvine, who followed 430 employees who lost their jobs with Illinois Bell when the company factory closed. He found that most of the workers suffered ill health effects from the crisis, but one-third were essentially unaffected. As the article states, one would assume that the one-third who fared well probably enjoyed "peaceful, privileged circumstances" outside the factory. In fact, however, this group shared in common relatively tumultuous childhoods. Maddi concluded that the adversity they faced in their early lives primed them for challenges later in life. The earlier stresses and subsequent physiological and psychological responses that were stored in their memories served to protect them from overreacting and compromising their general health and well-being.

Stress can protect us if we contextualize it positively. To a significant extent, we learn how to appropriate it through our early experiences. The *Newsweek* article cites a Stanford University study of baboons illustrating the connection between childhood experience and the ability to cope with stress. In the study, Dr. Robert Sapolsky discovered that baboon mothers that exhibited calm, controlled responses to stress nurtured in their male offspring the ability to choose only fights with other males that they were assured to win. Males that had no such role models became easily angered when confronted with challenges and often fought in an "insane" manner, often emerging less than victorious in their frequent scuffles. Furthermore, Sapolsky claims, the mothers of the more successful alpha-males were ones that allowed their young greater independence and control of their own actions. The implication for humans whose lives are full of stress are clear: Choose your battles wisely. And mothers, who today cope with multiple stressors, need to model positive behavior and allow their children to follow their own instincts when faced with fear so that they may integrate those important coping mechanisms.

A definitive line distinguishing a healthy from an unhealthy amount of stress is unclear, because so many variables exist in any given encounter with stress. But one point emerges from all the studies: People need to learn to manage the inevitable stress in their lives. They must recognize some of the symptoms of unhealthy stress—fatigue, irritability, sleep disorders, inability to focus, eating disorders, relationship problems, compromised immunity to illness—and adjust their lives to minimize these harmful effects. Staying calm in the face of a challenge is one way to thwart the consequences of stress and maximize the benefits of coping successfully with difficult situations. The fear of the consequences of stress only exacerbates the negative effects. We must accept that life is full of obstacles and that some stress is good. Learning to cope with it in a calm and reasonable manner can actually improve the quality of our lives. The ability to accept the challenge of adversity develops character and leadership, humility, common sense, and resourcefulness, allowing us to become survivors of the fittest in the evolutionary madness of life in the 21st century.

> "The greatest weapon against stress
> is our ability to choose one thought over another."
> —WILLIAM JAMES

A troubling quarrel with Tom over folding the laundry (of all trivial things!) made Michelle realize that she had to get her stress under control before it destroyed her marriage.

After the argument with Tom, she called her sister, Brenda, to discuss their mother's situation. Brenda was surprised to hear how stressed out Michelle sounded because Michelle always seemed so level-headed. Brenda agreed to help out more with their mother's care, and they started looking into options for hiring part-time nursing care. This would mean fewer out-of-town trips for Michelle, so she could spend more time with her own family and pay a little more attention to herself.

Then, Tom and Michelle started taking a walk together after dinner each evening. This time together allowed the couple to reconnect—and the fresh air and exercise really made them feel good, which, in turn, helped improve their relationship! Michelle also explained to Tom that her lack of sexual desire didn't mean she no longer loved him or craved his company. Tom agreed to help more around the house and with the children, and in doing so, he developed an appreciation for all she had been doing for their family. As Michelle reduced the tension in her life and as Tom became more of a partner in the relationship, she and Tom were both pleased to find themselves having sex more often!

Questions for Reflection

1. What events are causing stress in your life right now?

2. If you're under stress, what impact has this had on your libido? What about your partner's? Is there a discrepancy between your desire and your partner's?

3. What activities help you to feel better when you're under a great deal of stress? Have you been neglecting those activities lately?

4. What decisions do you need to make to resolve some of the stressful issues that have been impacting your life and libido?

5. What do you need from your partner to help deal with the sources of stress in your life? How will you communicate this to him in a nonconfrontational manner?

6. How might you use stress to benefit you? Can you learn to keep calm during those trying times? Can you model that behavior for others?

7. What are some ways you and your partner can work together to alleviate stress? Partner massage? Exercise together—tennis, golf, walking?

CHAPTER 7

FSD—The Female "Erectile Dysfunction"

"Sometimes we make love with our eyes. Sometimes we make love with our hands. Sometimes we make love with our bodies. Always we make love with our hearts."

—AUTHOR UNKNOWN

OVER THE PAST FOUR years, Anne, a 39-year-old mother of three and devoted wife to her husband, Michael, has lost just about all desire for any type of sexual intimacy. "I just can't figure out why," she said to me. "I'm happy with everything in my life, and my relationship with my husband overall is really good. Michael and I have talked about this, and I've reassured him it's not about him. And he's been so loving and sensitive in trying to help. He says I'm probably just stressed and overworked, so we've hired a housekeeper to come in once a week to help out with the housekeeping chores. He's encouraged me to join the gym and said that any time I want to get together with my friends, he'll make every effort to take the kids so I can have more time with them. He's even tried to do more of the 'little things,' such as holding my hand when we walk together and bringing me flowers more often. And just last night, he drew a bubble bath for me and placed a candle by the tub so I could just be alone and relaxed. It was so sweet!

"But even after all that, later in bed when he began to caress me, I started up with excuses to avoid sex—something I've been doing for the last six months. I've been coming to bed after Michael is asleep, intentionally slipping out of bed before he awakes, and I even let our kids have playtime and cuddle in our bed beyond their bedtime. Poor Michael! He can't figure out what has happened to his once amorous wife."

Concerned about her complete lack of desire and its potential effect on her relationship with Michael, Anne came to see me. "I sure hope you can help me!" she said. "I've heard of erectile dysfunction for men, but, in my case, I think I may have 'vaginal dysfunction,' or whatever is the equivalent of ED in women!"

Actually, the label Anne has given to her aversion to sex isn't too far off the mark. As the lead investigator in an international clinical trial investigating a new drug for treatment of decreased sexual desire in women, I have interviewed several hundred women with the same condition as Anne's. Through my study, I've been able to pinpoint some of the reasons some women avoid sexual intimacy altogether.

The clinical term for what Anne is going through is female sexual dysfunction, or FSD. This general term is used to describe certain conditions in which a woman may experience decreased sexual feelings, thoughts, fantasies, and lack of physical sensations with sexual activity.

This cumbersome term may sound like just another clinical term doctors might toss about at a medical conference, but it's worth your acknowledgment. When an OB/GYN uses the term FSD, it doesn't mean that the patient is simply suffering from low libido. Rather, she has reached a point of being completely unwilling, and sometimes unable, to respond to sexual activity, even when there exists great affection for her partner. When a doctor hears that a patient no longer willingly engages in activities such as caressing, foreplay, and vaginal intercourse, then there may be a true "clinical" dysfunction.

Unlike male sexual dysfunction, such as erectile dysfunction, which has a predominantly biological cause (lack of sufficient blood flow to achieve or maintain erection), in women the cause is more likely psychological. What this means is that we can give the little blue pill, Viagra, to men and see a phenomenal increase in their ability to perform, but these medications usually can't fix FSD—helping to increase vaginal blood flow will not necessarily help the female patient to "turn on."

After completing Anne's exam and interview, I diagnosed her with hypoactive sexual desire disorder, a condition marked by a complete absence of sexual desire. I ran blood tests to check her certain hormones and cholesterol levels (HDL/LDL and total cholesterol) and instructed her to apply one-eighth teaspoon of 2 percent testosterone gel to her inner wrist every morning. At Anne's five-week checkup with me, she told me that she felt "back to normal," and she and Michael were both delighted that their sex life had revived. Fortunately, Anne did not experience any negative side effects with the treatment, such as irritability, facial hair growth, or acne, which may occur. I will continue to see Anne in the office for checkups to monitor her blood cholesterol levels and make sure she goes in for her annual screening mammograms.

Anne's success with reclaiming her desire for sex supports the fact that women needn't settle for a low or absent libido and the consequential dissatisfaction it brings to them and their partner.

> *"Problems are not stop signs, they are guidelines."*
> —DR. ROBERT SCHULLER

Sexual Dysfunction and the Importance of an Accurate Diagnosis

The American Psychiatry Association has created four categories of female sexual dysfunction (listed below). Since these conditions have been getting the attention of medical professionals like myself, there has been much debate about whether to label them true "dysfunctions" or "disorders." While that debate rages on, the bottom line is that sexual intimacy is a vital part of our overall health, and when absent, it's a condition that now fortunately can be treated.

Although the four categories of female sexual dysfunction may appear similar to a layperson, an expert in the field of sexual medicine recognizes the subtle differences among them. And that fine line can help OB/GYNs and other health-care professionals better assess and thus treat their patients more accurately. Let me just add that before any doctor rushes to label a problem as sexual dysfunction, two elements must be present: time and distress. How long has the woman been having these symptoms, and to what extent are they compromising the quality of her life? A patient needs to tell me that she has been experiencing the symptoms for at least six months before I will diagnose FSD. Next, the woman needs to express that she is "distressed" or frustrated, unhappy, worried, bothered, or dissatisfied with her sex life. In the presence of these two elements—time and distress—the doctor or health-care professional can begin treatment for the problem.

So here are the four categories of sexual dysfunction and the distinctions among them:

1. Sexual Desire Disorders

Within this category, there are two sub-types:

- **Hypoactive sexual desire disorder (HSDD).** This is the most common condition that I see in my patients. Here, a woman will describe to me a lessening or absence of any desire for sex, experience a lack of sexual fantasies or thoughts about sex, and report a lack of being receptive to sexual activity. In making this diagnosis, I need to make sure that there are not any medical conditions, such as hypothyroidism or depression, that may account for her sexual complaints.

- **Sexual aversion disorder.** A patient with this disorder will do almost anything to disengage from all sexual contact with her partner. She does not enjoy sex or sexual intimacy. In fact, when she is confronted with sexual advances from her partner, she becomes anxious, fearful, and even disgusted. She makes conscious efforts to avoid sex—such as going to bed later than her partner or sleeping with the kids in the bed.

2. Female Sexual Arousal Disorder

Patients with this condition enjoyed sex when they first became active, then later become distressed because they are unable to become sexually excited, either mentally or physically, in situations like foreplay with a partner, self-stimulation (masturbation), or sexual fantasy. What before could make them all warm and tingly no longer can. A woman with this disorder can't seem to get any sexual feelings flowing, either in her head or her genital area. Because of this lack of mental and physical connection, she does not become lubricated, which leads to painful intercourse—which will cause her to pull farther away from wanting sexual intimacy.

3. Female Orgasmic Disorder

A patient with this disorder enjoys sexual intimacy but can't achieve orgasm. She can't seem to "let go" and release the physical and emotional obstacles that are holding her back. Over the years, I have had many women report a temporary inability to reach orgasm. Yet if a patient tells me that she cannot reach orgasm on a continuous basis for at least six months, I need to help investigate this problem with her.

4. Sexual Pain Disorders

- **Vaginismus.** I have diagnosed quite a few patients with this condition. On physical examination, when I am inserting a speculum, the patient involuntarily contracts the muscles in the lower one-third of her vagina. This unconscious vaginal muscle tightening can also occurs with tampon insertion, as well as with attempted penile penetration by her partner. Understandably, this again can cause much distress for both the patient and her partner.

- **Dyspaurenia.** A patient with this disorder has persistent or recurrent pain within the vaginal and genital area during sexual activity. This condition has become more and more common as more "baby boomers" are entering menopause and women are living longer than ever before. Patients report symptoms of sharp, cutting, "knife-like" pain with intercourse. They actually want to have sex, but due to their intolerable pain, they eventually dislike and shun sex with their partner. Other things besides menopause can lead to this condition, including scar tissue that develops after vaginal surgery or vaginal delivery of an infant, thinning of vaginal tissues in women who are breastfeeding, and allergic reactions to hygiene products. In addition to pain, these patients may experience itching, burning, and swelling in their genital area.

In my practice, there are certain screening tools to help diagnose patients and see whether they fit these conditions. I routinely ask a set of questions, some of which are included below, to determine whether they truly have a disorder or not.

Change in desire:
1. On a scale of 1 to 10 (10 being the highest), how would you rate your level of sexual desire or interest right now?

2. Is this a significant change from your previous level of desire?

3. Are you feeling troubled or frustrated by this decrease in sexual interest?

4. How often over the past two to three months have you thought about having sex or being physically intimate with your partner?

5. Have you had any dreams lately that were of a sexual nature?

Change in physical response:
1. Have you noticed that you are less aroused by things your partner is doing?

2. Have you noticed more difficulty in becoming lubricated?

3. Have you noticed more delay or inability to achieve orgasm?

4. Are you having any pain with sexual intimacy?

Potential reasons for this change:

1. What reasons do you believe might be accounting for this diminished desire?

2. Do you have any previously diagnosed or undiagnosed physical or psychological conditions that you believe might be involved? Are you and your partner having any problems in your present relationship, such as financial stresses or problems with child-rearing?

3. Have you or your partner ever been unfaithful, and if so, how has this changed your sexual relationship?

4. Are you noticing that you are drinking more than you used to? Do you believe you might have a drinking problem?

5. Are you using recreational drugs?

6. Are you taking any new medications that might be affecting your sexual interest?

7. Are you having any changes in your menstrual cycles? Mood swings or other hormonal changes that you feel might be contributing?

8. What is your level of desire when you are on vacation with your partner? Is it the same, or does it improve?

The answers to these questions are insightful, especially number eight. This last question provides a great deal of information for me as a diagnosing physician. If the patient answers that her level of desire and ability to "perform" improves when she and her partner take a weeklong romantic vacation, then she probably doesn't have any of the female sexual

Frequently Asked Question...

My husband has been taking Viagra and it has done wonders for his desire and sexual performance. Would there be any harm in taking half of one of his pills to see if it could help me?

If your partner's doctor diagnoses him with erectile dysfunction, he may be prescribed a medication such as Viagra. While this little blue pill has done wonders for men, it has not panned out to be a panacea for women. Many studies done over the years have found that it really didn't get women all revved up and craving sex. Chemical compounds—such as Viagra and other medications to treat erectile dysfunction—affect men's and women's libido differently. When Pfizer, the pharmaceutical company that makes Viagra, investigated the drug's effect on women, it was found to be beneficial only in certain situations, such as in women with neurological conditions such as diabetes or multiple sclerosis, and in women on antidepressants with decreased arousal.

For men, Viagra causes smooth muscle relaxation, which increases blood flow to the penis, allowing it to engorge and become erect. In women, the issue with decreased libido is not one of blood flow, or lack thereof; it really has to do with the main female sexual organ—the brain! So if you took half of your partner's pill, you might find that you feel some tingling or blood flow in your genital area, but this probably will not be enough to get you "in the mood" because many factors are involved in a woman's desire, which is the focus of this book.

dysfunction disorders mentioned above. If her level remains low even during a relaxing getaway with her sexual partner, then I delve more deeply into which of the above conditions she may have.

"Sex is a discovery." —FANNIE HURST

Treatment Options for
Female Sexual Dysfunction

So let's say that you have come to me and we have determined that indeed you are suffering from one of the conditions. Now what? Luckily, for many of these, there are readily available solutions. For the others, more research needs to be done to help women.

Vaginal dryness and pain with intercourse. To get the vagina the adequate lubrication for sex not to hurt, I initially recommend lubricants. Some of my patients' favorites are Replense and Astroglide.

If lubricants do not work to make sex more comfortable, I prescribe vaginal estrogen therapy, which comes in three different forms: vaginal cream, vaginal tablets, and a vaginal ring. I like to give my patients a choice as to which of these they prefer and that fits best into their lifestyle.

Problems with arousal and desire. We've all seen the commercials! Men become elated and literally jump with joy that they have found a pill to boost getting and maintaining an erection. When Viagra was first launched in March 1998, it blazed the trail for treating men with sexual dysfunction, specifically for those who had problems with erectile dysfunction. So why hasn't it shown to be such a trailblazer for women?

Viagra works by inhibiting a certain enzyme (Phosphodiesterase-5) that causes production of high levels of nitrous oxide. Nitrous oxide increases blood flow to the genital tissues (vagina and penis). This shunting of blood to the penis allows men to become erect and maintain the erection. In women, the deluge of increased blood to the vaginal tissues will allow them to become engorged and relaxed. Well, so what if there's more blood down there? This increase in blood to the area below her waistline (her genitals) doesn't solve the problem of the complex control panel above her belt—her brain! In women, the most important organ for desire is the brain, not the genital tissues. If a woman is not excited, interested, or aroused by certain stimuli, no amount of increased blood flow to her genital area will make a difference.

However, in certain women, such as those suffering from diabetes or multiple sclerosis, improvement with Viagra has been shown, as both of these conditions involve the element of blood flow to the vaginal tissues. One other group that showed benefit with use of the "little blue pill" were women diagnosed with depression who were taking selective serotonin reuptake inhibitors (SSRIs) and having difficulty with orgasm.[1] The important message to take away from all of this is that Viagra is not the panacea for women that it is for men. Although some women have reported to me a benefit with its use, this may be a placebo effect, or possibly a true effect from bloodflow increasing arousal. Viagra is not currently available for use in women, and if a physician prescribes it for you, this would be considered an "off-label" use that needs to be thoroughly discussed before starting. Keep in mind that Viagra's use for women has not been thoroughly tested in clinical trials. The female brain and its triggers for arousal are very different—in general, no amount of increased blood flow using Viagra is going to help.

> *"Sexual love is the most stupendous fact of the universe,*
> *and the most magical mystery our poor blind senses know."*
> —AMY LOWELL

Good News for the Future

As a researcher in women's libido, I'm always on the lookout for new ways to improve women's lives, and especially their overall issues with libido. What I see now is that pharmaceutical companies are pouring millions of dollars into research and development, all trying to find the "wonder drug" to spark a woman's desire. Several prescription drugs are currently undergoing clinical trials. Here are four that show promise for "lighting the fire."

Bremelanotide *(Palatin Technologies)*: Bremelanotide was originally tested as a sunless tanning agent that was inhaled through the nose. Test showed that it also caused sexual arousal and spontaneous erections in men. Unfortunately, the trials also demonstrated increased blood pressure in patients, so further studies were abandoned in 2007. Palatin Technologies decided to try a different route of delivery, by injection. There was no evidence of blood pressure elevation, so Palatin is now in discussion with the FDA to resume Phase II studies in both erectile dysfunction (ED) and female sexual dysfunction (FSD).

Femprox *(NexMed, Inc.)*: Femprox is a topical cream containing alprostadil, a vasodilator that causes the blood vessels to dilate. Applied prior to sex in the genital area, it has been shown to increase sexual arousal in premenopausal and postmenopausal women. Alprostadil is currently approved in the United States as a urethral suppository for erectile dysfunction in men. Initial studies of Femprox were conducted in China and Hong Kong, where it is now readily available. NexMed is presently seeking FDA approval in the U.S.

Libigel *(BioSante Pharmaceuticals)*: This drug is a transdermal testosterone gel (300 micrograms) being studied to get Food and Drug Administration approval for treating decreased desire in women. This study involves women who have undergone surgical menopause (removal of the ovaries) and are using estrogen therapy for the treatment of menopausal symptoms. The company making Libigel is hoping to finalize data collection in the next one to two years, at which time the FDA will then evaluate their results and determine whether they require further data, such as safety with regard to breast cancer and cardiovascular disease.

Flibanserin *(Boehringer-Ingelheim)*: This drug works at the serotonin receptor sites and was serendipitously found to improve sexual desire in women who were being studied for depression. Initial clinical trials in 1992 showed that women studied noticed fewer depressive symptoms as well as increased sexual thoughts and desire. Clinical trials are presently being conducted in the United States, including at my own research site, Pacific Coast Research Center, with hope for FDA approval in early 2010.

Many of my patients do not necessarily want to take prescription drugs and ask me about "natural" or herbal remedies. These remedies have not undergone FDA testing or clinical trials to investigate their safety or determine their efficacy. Nevertheless, many women do want some options. Below are some herbal remedies that a significant number of my patients have reported to me as helping to stimulate their interest in sexual intimacy and physical sensations with sexual activity.

Argin-Max *(Daily Wellness Company)*: Argin-Max is an herbal formulation that contains an amino acid, L-arginine, that increases nitric oxide production, blood flow, and blood vessel dilation. This remedy contains other vitamins and minerals, including gingko biloba (which enhances blood flow) and ginseng (a mild stimulant). Two formulations are available: one for men and one for women. The women's formula also contains damiana, an herb known to calm and help decrease anxiety. In clinical trials over a four-week period, improvement in sexual desire was seen in women taking the herbal formulation.

Vigorelle *(Advanced Botanicals)*: Vigorelle topical cream has for many patients allowed them to "feel" more in the genital area. one Some describe their experience with sexual activity prior to using this cream as "muffled," but after applying it they had more "tingling." This is most likely due to the menthol contained in this cream, along with the other components, L-arginine HCL, damiana leaf, organic wild yam, gingko biloba, and peppermint leaf.

Testosterone for Women: Is It Worth the Risk?

A woman produces 50 percent less testosterone at age 40 than she did at age 20. So does this depleted hormone level really affect a woman's desire for sex? The answer is yes. The decline in testosterone definitely has an impact on desire, leading to a marked decrease in her thoughts of, interest in, or initiation of steamy moments with her partner. Many of my patients have asked me, "Why not just give me more testosterone so I'll be back to the amount I had in my early twenties?"

The answer is not necessarily that easy. Studies have shown a significant benefit to adding testosterone for women with decreased desire[2] and for those with low normal levels of testosterone. Using testosterone may help rev up your libido but it also might cause you some unwanted side effects, such as increased facial hair, irritability, and acne. That is why it is so important that you team with your physician to determine the correct dose for you and monitor you for any of these side effects.

Presently, there are different forms of testosterone that I prescribe to my patients. An oral combination of testosterone with estrogen, known as Estratest, is currently available and is approved by the FDA. I also use the help of my compounding pharmacist to compound specific testosterone creams and gels for my patients. These require a physician's order and are not approved by the FDA, yet are presently used "off label" by many gynecologists, endocrinologists, and anti aging experts. Gels and creams are applied to the inner wrist. In general, it takes at least three to four weeks before any benefit is seen. I usually have my patients come back in four to five weeks after starting testosterone treatment to see how they are doing. If they hug me and say they and their husband love me for helping out their sex life, I am happy. If no increase in desire to connect is seen, I may consider slightly increasing their dose as long as no other side effects are occurring.

It is also important to remember that with any medication, there are risks as well as benefits. With testosterone therapy, some studies have shown an increase in breast cancer and stroke.[3] Thus it is essential that you discuss any risk factors with your physician and that you that undergo certain blood tests to check cholesterol levels, assess risk for heart disease, and have regular mammograms or breast screening.

I have seen how FSD can be devastating to women as well as to their intimate relationships. The first step in helping a woman is to understand exactly what problem she is having and why. By carefully gleaning through all of the information that a patient gives me, I can then see how her level of self-esteem, severity of life stresses, physical and hormonal changes, difficult relationship issues, as well as other factors all tie together. By revealing her symptoms to me and being open with her part-ner, a woman who has FSD can get help, explore the possible obstacles, and allow for better understanding and fulfillment in her life.

Questions for Reflection

1. Have you spoken with your physician about your lack of desire? If not, what factors are preventing you from doing so?

2. Are your symptoms causing you "distress"? Have they lasted more than six months?

3. Reading through the four classifications of sexual dysfunction in this chapter, which one do you feel might apply to you?

4. Take a close look at the list of questions I have included in this chapter and answer them as honestly as possible.

5. Would you consider taking a medication to increase your libido?

6. Would you consider taking herbal treatments or using a non–FDA-approved treatment?

CHAPTER 8

Medications and Health Conditions that Can Shelve Your Libido

"Health is a state of complete harmony of the body, mind and spirit. When one is free from physical disabilities and mental distractions, the gates of the soul open."
—B. K. S. IYENGAR

DONNA IS A 26-YEAR-OLD single woman in a relatively new relationship with Steve. She came to my office to discuss her contraceptive options and decided on the birth control pill. But after three months on the pill, Donna's libido plummeted—not something that usually happens to a healthy woman of 26! Since it didn't appear to be a psychological or relationship issue, we discussed the fact that the birth control pill, as well as other hormonal contraceptive regimens (the patch and the ring), may cause a decrease in desire for some women. We talked about other options, and I suggested that Donna switch to a form of birth control that did not contain hormones, and that she make a follow-up appointment so we could evaluate whether switching "medications" better served her.

When I saw Donna three months later, she reported that she was doing well with her birth control, and that her libido was "healthy and happy."

Certain Medications Sedate Your Love Life

Are you surprised to learn that both prescription and nonprescription medications can alter sexual desire, arousal, and orgasm? They can. Be sure to continue taking all prescribed medicines as your doctor instructed you, but if you find that your sexual desire and/or performance has changed several weeks after beginning a new medication, talk to your doctor to see whether there is a different medication you might try, one that won't send your libido packing.

Some medications interfere with libido by affecting the following:

■ Hormonal levels of estrogen and testosterone

■ Neurological/brain function (antidepressants and anti-anxiety medications that change levels of neurotransmitters, sedatives, and mood stabilizers)

■ Blood flow (such as antihypertensives)

Levels of estrogen and testosterone are extremely important as a stimulus for increased thoughts of and desire for sex. As mentioned in Chapter 4, neurotransmitters are also important for sexual desire. Dopamine increases sexual function, whereas serotonin decreases sexual function. And any medication that affects blood flow can impact the arousal/excitement phase in women (and erection in men). Here are some categories of drugs that affect libido:

■ Lipid-/cholesterol-lowering drugs

■ Thyroid, adrenal, and other hormone regulators

■ Gastrointestinal medications

■ Antihistamines/cold medications

The following table lists of some of the most common medications that affect libido. It is important to remember that not all of these drugs will cause low libido in everyone, since each individual reacts differently to medications. I always ask my patients if they have experienced any decrease in libido in the past, and whether or not they were taking any specific medications at that time. If you are taking a medication that might be affecting your libido, consider various options, including lowering the dose or finding a different type of medication for the same condition that might have fewer side effects.

Are you taking any of these—or other—medications in the following categories?

Allergy medications

Hormonal contraceptives
    Birth-control pill, patch, and ring

Anti-hypertensives for treatment of high blood pressure
    ACE inhibitors
    Alpha blockers
    Beta blockers
    Calcium channel blockers
    Clonidine
    Diuretics
    Methyldopa

Cholesterol-lowering medications
    Statins
    Fibrates

Medications for gastrointestinal disorders
    Cimetidine
    Metoclopramide
    Omeprazole

Medications for neurological conditions
    Anticonvulsants
    Antidepressants
    Anti-epileptics
    Antihistamines
    Anti-Parkinson's medicines
    Benzodiazepines
    Narcotics for pain control

Anti-cancer medications

Chemotherapy drugs for treatment of any type of cancer

If you or your partner are taking medications for any of the above conditions and are experiencing sexual side effects, please speak with your
doctor. In my practice, I frequently consider and prescribe alternatives
that do not affect the libido, at least not to the extent that the other
medications may. If your medication is the only one available to treat a
specific condition and is critical to you or your partner's health, then I
would discuss ways to enhance sex without changing the medication. For
instance, you might be more creative and playful and more adventurous
in finding ways to pleasure each other—such as by experimenting with
various sex toys or trying a new exotic lubricant. Vibrators can enhance
foreplay and stimulate arousal, and so on.

   Still, even with trying new things, it is important to realize that certain
medications can have a negative impact on arousal or achieving orgasm.
This means that you or your partner may need more "warm-up" time or
time to reach orgasm. Be patient, and use this time as an opportunity to
connect with each other—in spite of the negative effects of the medication on your libido.

> *"It is easy to get a thousand prescriptions*
> *but hard to get one single remedy."* —CHINESE PROVERB

Antidepressants

Unfortunately, depression itself can shoot down your libido, and antidepressant medications don't usually help matters within the sexual arena.
Your doctor may have prescribed antidepressants for you to stay on course
and enjoy life, but some antidepressants may further lower desire and
block the ability to achieve sexual satisfaction. They are, in fact, one of
the most common causes of decreased libido. If you are being treated for
depression, closely follow your doctor's orders about specific dosing and

Frequently Asked Question...

My husband recently was diag-nosed with prostate cancer. Am I at any risk of developing cancer because of this? No, you are not at any risk of developing cancer by having sex together. In fact, women can help decrease the risk of prostate cancer in their partners by having regular sexual relations. Studies have shown that men who have frequent ejaculations have a lesser risk of developing prostate cancer.

timing of medications. If you feel something is still not quite right, be open with your physician and inquire about alternative medications or other supplemental treatments that might decrease these unwanted effects. Of course, if your doctor does not see the importance of your concerns, then you may choose to get a second opinion, finding someone who may be more attentive to your case and may have more expertise in this area.

Many people are on antidepressants for months and even years, and so the persistently decreased libido can undermine the sexual satisfaction of the couple. It has been my experience that many patients suffering from clinical depression are not sure whether their lack of sex drive is a result of their antidepressant or their depression.

If you are on any of the following commonly used medications for depression and anxiety and you are experiencing sexual side effects, speak to your doctor. You should not have to make compromises with your health and happiness:

- Antidepressants: Prozac, Zoloft, Paxil, Luvox, Serzone, BuSpar, Norpramin, Prolixin, Lithium, Mellaril, Nardil, Serax, Anafranil, Elavil, Tofranil, Sinequan, Pamelor

- Mood Stabilizers/Neuroleptics: Thorazine, Haldol, Zyprexa

- Sedatives: Librium, Valium, Xanax, Quaalude (methaqualone), Barbiturates, Ativan

You may not need a medical lecture on the physiology of taking these medications, but you should know why they kill libido. In short, selective serotonin reuptake inhibitors, a classification of drugs known as SSRIs, are commonly used to treat depression, premenstrual syndrome, and anxiety. Unfortunately, they frequently cause sexual dysfunction in both men and women.

When my patients are having symptoms of depression and need to be on an antidepressant, we work together to find the medication that will best treat their depression while having the least negative effect on their sexual desire, especially regarding their ability to become aroused or reach orgasm. To better address these consequences to a patient's libido, I frequently ask the following questions:

■ Have you experienced any sexual difficulties?

■ Have you noticed that you're more apathetic toward having sex?

■ Have you experienced any difficulty with "getting in the mood"?

■ Have you noticed any decrease in lubrication?

■ Have you experienced a delay in reaching orgasm?

■ Have you seen a complete lack of ability to complete orgasm?

After a patient has started on any of these medications or been on one for a period of time, I have her follow up with me to see how she is responding to the treatment. I also ask whether she is noticing any improvement in her depression or anxiety and if she is experiencing any new symptoms, especially in the sexual arena. If so, she and I work together to find the best medication to keep her depression at bay but her libido sailing smoothly.

Four Ways to Light a Fire
Under Your Libido

Studies have found that people who are taking antidepressants such as Zoloft may be literally depressing their chances of falling in love. According to biological anthropologist Helen Fisher and psychiatrist James Thomson, who specialize in studies of romantic attachment, "anti-depressants alter brain chemistry in a way that minimizes the chance of falling in love."[1] The most significant potential consequence of serotonin blockers like Zoloft occurs when they affect dopamine levels in the brain. As you recall, serotonin is the hormone that helps to govern mood but can also lead to decreased desire and ability to become aroused. In general, dopamine is the hormone that fuels impulse and makes us feel that romantic "rush" when we see our beloved. To read more about the brain chemistry of these important hormones, see Chapter 4.

If you are experiencing sexual side effects from antidepressants, it is critical that you disclose them to your doctor so you can work together to find the best answer for you. Again, do not stop any medication or change any part of your regimen without first discussing this with your physician. Here are some ways I treat women who want to light the fire under their libido. As always, check with your doctor to see if s/he agrees this is the best course of action for you.

1. Take a "drug holiday." With advice from your doctor, stop taking the medication for a certain amount of time or have certain days when you don't take the medication. For instance, a "weekend holiday" would involve stopping the medication after the Thursday morning dose and resuming the next dose on Sunday. This "holiday" will lead to decreased levels of medication in your body. This may be wonderful for your libido but dangerous for your depression/anxiety, so I tread very gently with this option, as I do not want to put my patients at any undue risk for increased anxiety or depressive symptoms. Some medications are metabolized in your body very quickly, allowing better sexual response without a marked change in mood benefits. Other medications have extremely long half-lives (the time for medication to be metabolized to 50 percent of its initial therapeutic dose), so a short interruption in treatment may have no effect at all and prove not to be helpful. Other anti-depressant medications, which have a very short half-life, may show no benefit in desire but an actual decrease in efficacy for treating depression. Be sure to speak with your physician before stopping any medications.

2. Change the medication. I have found that changing the type of medication a patient is on can significantly benefit her in reducing sexual side effects. Another way to help counteract the negative impact of certain medications is to add a second medication. One that I commonly use is Bupropion (Wellbutrin), as it has been shown to have the fewest, if any, sexual side effects and may be used in addition to or in place of an SSRI.

3. Change the dose of medication. Many times, I have seen that the dosage of an antidepressant can be lowered without changing the benefit in treatment of depression and help decrease the negative impact on sexual desire. It is always wise to use the lowest effective dosage of a drug.

4. Consider herbal remedies. Patients who tell me they are sure that taking antidepressants creates a disinterest in sex can sometimes find relief in taking herbs in addition to their antidepressant regimen or trying natural therapies as a sole treatment. Before adding an herbal remedy or completely changing over to one, consult with your health-care professional.

Herbs have been used for their therapeutic value since the dawn of humankind to promote health, well-being, and an energetic sex life. Many herbs can effectively battle depression without unwanted side effects. Scientific evidence supports the benefits of herbs for increasing sexual urge and pleasure. In fact, up to 25 percent of modern medicines are based on products derived from plant origins. Herbs that have been shown to enhance libido include the following:

■ Maca

■ Saw palmetto

- Passion flower

- Ginseng

- Wild lettuce leaf

These herbs work to set the mood, increase sexual desire and drive, increase sexual pleasure, and boost energy levels. They have also been found to treat health conditions that can inhibit sex, such as impotence, prostate problems, menopause, PMS, and arthritis. Again, always speak to your health-care provider before starting any herbal remedy.

"The yoga mat is a good place to turn when talk therapy and antidepressants aren't enough." —AMY WEINTRAUB

Contraceptives

As Donna found, hormone-containing contraceptives, such as the pill, the patch, and the ring, are sometimes associated with decreased libido, arousal disorder, and vaginal dryness in women. These effects occur because the majority of hormonal contraceptive methods (combined synthetic estrogens and synthetic progestins) are designed to prevent pregnancy by interfering with the ovaries' ability to ovulate, leading to hormonal changes. Specifically, these decrease the production of certain hormones called androgens, such as testosterone, a decrease that directly influences sex drive and pleasure.

A second reason for less sexual "mo-jo" is that these combined hormonal birth-control methods increase the production of a protein called sex-hormone binding globulin (SHBG). This protein, which binds to the free hormones circulating in your bloodstream, makes them ineffective within your tissues. Think of Pac-man-type proteins that bind to available targets. When the number of SHBG Pac-man particles increases, the free hormone testosterone becomes less available to fuel desire. Studies have shown a link between high levels of SHBG and decreased sexual desire.[2]

This is not the type of birth control most patients are seeking!

If you are on any type of combined hormonal contraceptive (the pill, the patch, or the ring) and are experiencing lowered libido, speak to your health-care provider to see whether there are any viable alternatives for you. There are forms of contraception that do not contain synthetic hormones and may have less negative impact on your "urge to merge." These alternative birth-control methods include barrier methods, such as condoms or diaphragms, and intrauterine contraception (such as the Paragard IUD and Mirena IUS).

> *"Condoms aren't completely safe.*
> *A friend of mine was wearing one and got hit by a bus."*
> —Bob Rubin

Hormone Therapy (HT)

The use of hormone therapy for treatment of menopausal symptoms has become extremely controversial. Many physicians oppose the use of hormone therapy for their patients, while the majority of OB/GYN physicians tend to advocate its use, at least in the short term, for alleviating the unwanted hot flashes, night sweats, and decreased libido associated with menopause.

The key here is the route and timing of administration of the therapeutic hormones. Oral medications can decrease the availability of testosterone via levels of SHBG, as discussed above, which can lead to decreased desire in women. Transdermal (through the skin) medications tend to cause fewer symptoms of decreased desire because they do not lead to a marked increase in SHBG, leading to higher circulating levels of free testosterone and more desire.

Over my 15 years of clinical research experience and private practice, I have closely witnessed the benefit of hormone therapy in my patients, in both the short and long terms. And, as lead investigator in trials established for the study of hot flashes and vaginal dryness, I have seen that these therapies greatly assist in creating the best treatment plans for my

Frequently Asked Question...

My hormones are all over the map, and I'm so tired of being controlled by them. What can I do if I don't want to take hormone therapy?

Certain lifestyle changes can definitely help keep your hormones under control. Dietary changes, such as switching from a high-fat, refined-carbohydrate diet to one containing more organic, raw, and unprocessed, low-fat foods has been shown to bring estrogen levels within a more normal range. Through an enzymatic reaction in our fatty tissue, adrenal steroids are converted into fat. The more fat you take in and the higher amount of fatty tissue that you have in your body, the higher the rate of conversion of androgen to estrogen, resulting in higher estrogen levels. Decreasing the amount of fat in your diet can therefore help in balancing your hormone levels, as well as decreasing your risk for heart disease.

patients. Daily, patients consult with me, vehemently complaining (and understandably so) about their severe hot flashes, night sweats, irritability, and lack of sexual desire. Many go on to add that they experience severe pain with sexual intimacy because of their vaginal dryness. In these situations, it is imperative that I have an intense, face-to-face conversation with my patient, explaining the pros and cons of hormone therapy. Hormone therapy may not be for everyone, but it definitely can help the patient who feels as though she is no longer in control of her emotional health. If you feel that you are about to tear your partner's head off and want nothing to do with sex, it may be time for a little HT help!

Overall, hormone therapy has been found to increase libido in menopausal women. Yet, as with all medications, there are risks and benefits—this is why it is important to speak with your doctor, discuss your symptoms, and manifest the best medical treatment plan as possible. Specifically, the benefits of hormone therapy include marked reduction in hot flashes, night sweats, and irritability. Much of this is due to the significantly improved sleep it promotes, with fewer early morning

Frequently Asked Question...

Is there such a thing as a "male menopause"? Some physicians specializing in anti-aging medicine do believe in this phenomenon and call it "andropause." In women, menopause causes a steep decline in the production of estrogen, sometimes leading to many side effects, such as hot flashes, sleep disturbances, mood swings, and irritability. Men, too, experience a decline in hormones, specifically testosterone, but this is a far more gradual process. Your partner may seem less vigorous, less stuck on thinking about sex, and less likely to initiate. This may be a completely normal progression for him, yet if it is distressing to your relationship, be open to discussing this with your partner and go together to his doctor for an evaluation.

awakenings and the ability to fall back asleep much faster. Yet, with these benefits come risks that include a higher rate of cardiovascular disease (stroke and heart attack) as well as breast cancer.[3] In general, the overall present consensus among medical professionals is for you to use the lowest effective dose for the shortest duration of time. Before jumping into or completely writing off hormone therapy, be sure to weigh the risks and benefits with your physician. Make sure that your physician is up to date on the most recent research and has a close pulse on the best forms of medications available. Only through this can you and your physician make the most appropriate, healthy decision for you.

"To control your hormones is to control your life." — BARRY SEARS

Health Conditions that Fizzle Desire

Good general health and well-being is essential for a fully functioning libido. Your first concern in achieving healthy sexuality and overall wellness should be those health issues that may compromise the quality of life and daily functioning and those that may even be life-threatening. Some of these conditions include the following:

Heart Disease

Research has shown a significant link between heart disease and decreased libido. Essentially, when heart disease prohibits adequate blood flow throughout the body and brain, you feel generally sluggish and often depressed. If you are already depressed, the physical and emotional stress of heart disease can cause serious problems, not the least of which occur in the bedroom. In order to promote a happy, energetic sex life, it is vital that women take care of their heart health.

There are many things we can do to minimize heart disease and ensure a vibrant sex life, such as:

- Exercise.

- Reduce your stress. Use meditation, yoga, or counseling to minimize and manage stress.

- Eat a diet that is low in bad cholesterol (found in red meat) and high in good fats (such as linseeds and hempseeds) and omega 3 fatty acids (such as salmon).

- Floss regularly. Maintaining optimum oral and gum health is linked to a healthy heart!

- Eat plenty of vital nutrients and antioxidants from fruits and vegetables.

- Practice forgiveness. Improved emotional and physical wellness can lead to a healthier heart. Practicing nonjudgment and tolerance are key to enjoying a happy heart and a vibrant sex life.

■ Breathe. Learn proper breathing techniques, which have been shown to lower blood pressure naturally.

Diabetes

Due to high blood sugar levels in patients with diabetes, there can be blood vessel damage to various organs. Studies have shown that women with diabetes may experience increased sexual dysfunction (problems with arousal and orgasm) and decreased sexual desire. If you have diabetes, it is imperative that you monitor your blood sugar levels very closely with your physician. This is also true for your partner! Recent studies have shown an association between diabetes, erectile dysfunction, and heart disease.[4] These problems are associated with blood vessel damage to the heart and genital organs. If your partner is experiencing any problems with erectile dysfunction, this may be a signal of future health problems—and a time for him to visit his doctor for a complete physical examination and laboratory evaluation.

Insomnia and Lack of Restful Sleep

Would you sometimes rather just take a nap than have sex with your partner? Do you feel exhausted by the end of the day? Or even at the start of the day? Sleep deprivation is a definite libido killer. Studies have shown that women who are happy in their marriages have more restful sleep compared to those women in less happy marriages.[5] The happier married women reported less difficulty falling asleep, less early morning awakening, and better ability to fall back asleep if awakened. According to their findings, being happy in your marriage may present benefits for sleep that go far beyond being a "happy" or "well-adjusted" person. Get the rest you need, and you and your partner will have more energy for sexual intimacy.

Many other medical conditions not included in the list can have a direct impact on your libido. Lifestyle factors such as excessive use of tobacco, alcohol, or illicit drugs can also affect libido in both men and women. For an average woman, excessive alcohol would mean an average of more than one drink per day (one beer, four to five ounces of wine, or one shot of hard liquor). Smoking cigarettes has been shown to be detrimental to overall health and increase risk of heart disease. For men, it has been shown that the greater number of cigarettes per day smoked, the greater the risk of heart attack and erectile dysfunction. Use of marijuana has been shown to decrease sperm production and function. It is also important to remember that women metabolize drugs and alcohol differently than men. A small amount of alcohol or illicit drugs can have a huge effect on a woman and her desire despite its having very little effect on her partner. If you're experiencing sexual dysfunction or a decrease in desire, it's important to mention any health conditions as well as lifestyle habits to your doctor. There could be a connection.

Libido is a complex function. Many factors affect its functioning, some to a significant extent, some to a lesser one. This chapter just briefly touches on the medications and health conditions that can affect desire. If you or your partner are experiencing any type of medical condition and/or taking any kind of medication and are experiencing decreased libido, talk to your doctor. There may well be an explanation for the problem for which your doctor can provide a simple solution.

Questions for Reflection

1. Are you on contraceptives, antidepressants, or any of the other medications listed in this chapter? If so, have you discussed their impact on your libido with your physician?

2. Do you have a chronic health condition, such as heart disease? Are you doing all you can to keep the disease under control and increase your sex drive?

3. If you're experiencing diminished libido, it could be the result of a medical condition. Have you had a physical recently? What habits (poor diet, smoking, etc.) might be negatively impacting your health and/or sexual desire?

4. What positive habits can you acquire (exercise, changing diet, etc.) that will improve your health and libido?

CHAPTER 9

Heart to Heart:
Using Communication to
Resuscitate Your Libido

"For women, the best aphrodisiacs are words. The G-spot
is in the ears. He who looks for it below there is wasting his time."
— ISABEL ALLENDE

WHEN MEGAN CAME TO my office for her annual exam, I could sense that something was troubling her. I asked her how things were going, and she quipped, "Except for my love life, everything is good!" With a bit of prompting, she told me about something that happened the evening before. The moment dinner was over, her husband got up and went to the TV room, while she was stuck in the kitchen...this was just the beginning of work around the house. She felt like crying. She had been running around since she came home from work, and all she had been thinking about was a warm bath and bed. She thought to herself, "Why doesn't it dawn on him to help me clean up so that I can have some down time, too?" Said Megan, "Unfortunately, not even giving him the silent treatment and cold shoulder got any help from him!"

"How good is Dan at reading your mind?" I asked. Megan grinned slightly and said, "Not very." I then asked her how long she and Dan had been creating this communication gap—and why. Megan had no immediate answer, realizing that their communication problem had been growing for a long time. And their relationship was not going to improve if they continued communicating—or not communicating—this way.

Megan admitted, "I guess we're both were pretty dissatisfied with the way we relate to one another, but we're just used to it. Oh well, I guess I should just be happy he comes home for dinner and isn't running around with his buddies instead!"

Does this problem sound familiar? Do you feel like you and your partner aren't really asking for and getting what you need from each other? Communication is essential in all aspects of our lives. Throughout this book, I have emphasized the importance of communication—the critical need to be honest with yourself and your partner. Learning to relate to one another in a loving manner is crucial to having a positive and loving relationship—which in turn is essential for maintaining a healthy sex life between you.

How would you assess your ability to communicate about your relationship? Ask yourself:

- How well do I communicate with my partner? Are we making time to talk things out?

- What am I communicating to my partner through my actions?

- How will I know that things are moving in the right direction?

- Am I unhappy about anything in my present relationship?

- What am I hoping to change about my relationship?

Now consider how your relationship is affecting your libido. Communicating their wants and needs regarding their sexual relationship is especially difficult for many people. Consider each of the following questions and discuss your answers with your partner. Encourage him to answer the questions also.

- Do we talk about sex?

- What sex acts turn me on? What about my partner?

- Do I look forward to sex with my partner?

- How do I rate our foreplay?

- How do I rate his ability to stimulate me?

- How do I respond to his advances?

- What would I like for him to *say* to get me interested in sex?

- What would I like him to do differently?

- When does our discussion of sex stop? What are we reluctant to say?

- What are the specific things he does or says that draw me away from him?

- What will be one of the first signs that my sex drive is getting back on track?

- What things will my partner notice about me when my passion returns?

- What three changes in my sexual health would I most like to bring about?

- What three things do I most like about my sexual self?

- What two things do I like least?

- Do I feel I have the skills to communicate my wants, needs, and desires with my partner?

- If my communication skills are lacking, do I lack the *desire* to communicate, or the skills to tell my partner what I want and need from our sexual relationship?

- What do I like most about having sex with my partner?

■ What do I like the least about having sex with my partner?

Over my 15 years of clinical practice, I have come to understand the impact that communication has on a couple's relationship and their sex life. Women so often refrain from saying what is really on their minds, or they sometimes play games—such as Megan did. While games such as "read my mind" or "the silent treatment" speak volumes, neither is likely to improve your life or your relationship.

Additionally, when your partner does or says something that disturbs you, keeping your feelings about it to yourself can be extremely destructive to your relationship. You may have tried in the past to tell your partner about your concerns, but if he didn't acknowledge your feelings or change his behavior, you may have simply resigned yourself to living with your unmet needs. Not saying what you mean or meaning what you say only causes frustration, leading to a simmering of negative energy that eventually explodes into fights, extramarital affairs, separation, or even divorce.

Over weeks, months, and years, these bottled-up feelings magnify to the point where the smallest problems may become insurmountable. You'll build walls in hopes of protecting yourself, but these same walls will block communication and the expression of love and intimacy. These emotional burdens may also, in fact, negatively affect your physical health.

"Self-expression must pass into communication for its fulfillment."
—PEARL S. BUCK

Eight Skills to Revive Communication

Men and women don't think alike. Communication between the sexes, therefore, does not come naturally, since men and women frequently have different styles of communicating. To stay connected, to stay in love, and to create an ongoing desire to stay in a harmonious and intimate relationship, couples need to exercise patience and persistence. They

Frequently Asked Question...

Our sex life has become so boring. How can we spice things up in the bedroom?
It is very common to fall into a rut in many aspects of your life, especially on the sexual front. You or your partner may be devoting too little time and effort to making sex fun and playful again. But you need to! If the thrill factor in your sex life has pretty much hit rock bottom, think of your five senses: touch, smell, taste, hearing, and sight. Love can be expressed with just a simple touch. How do you want your partner to touch you? How and where do you want to be caressed? There are plenty of erogenous zones, both below and above the waist! Learn the art of sensual massage, buy some new massage oils, and use feathers or ice cubes to bring out the tactile pleasures. Buy some fragrant candles with soft light, wear a spicy, alluring perfume, and put on some soft "mood music." Treat yourself to some sexy lingerie that might stretch your comfort zone a bit. Try role-playing and acting out playful fantasies. Take charge in bed   initiate—this will be welcomed by your partner.

The bottom line is being present, being self aware and aware of your partner. Step out of the "habit energy"; let go of distractions and challenges. Free yourself from self-doubt, harsh criticism, and distracting worries. This is a time for you! This will lead to further emotional, spiritual, and physical deepening.

have to create circumstances—the environment and the language—that will facilitate open communication. In short, couples have to work hard at communicating effectively.

The following suggestions will help you and your partner learn how to better listen to each other, acknowledge what is said, and openly discuss the issues in your relationship.

1. Arrange for time to talk. Choose a time for discussion when you both can focus on the issues. Don't try to talk to your partner about serious issues when he's trying to go to sleep or is absorbed in a football game! Agree to certain ground rules: Respect each other's opinions, even if you don't agree with them. Listen with an open heart and do not be defensive. Keep your goal in mind: to speak honestly, to listen open-mindedly, and to be heard. Make sure that both you and your partner have sufficient time to express your feelings without distractions or time restraints.

2. Keep growing your communications skills. Read books and articles about communication. Enlist a good coach or counselor. Listen to your partner in the same way that you would like him to listen to you. One great tool to use is a communication stick. Choose an object that you can pass back and forth. The person who holds the object is the only one who is allowed to speak.

3. Be an active listener. While the physical act of hearing—sound waves passing into the auditory canal—may be occurring, the more refined process of listening is a matter of the heart. Active listening means that one person speaks at a time, without interruption, criticism, or judgment. Then the listener acknowledges what the speaker has verbalized, paraphrasing what has been stated. This allows both parties to check that the meaning was communicated and confirm understanding.

4. Focus on only one point at a time. As we know, women are much more adept at multitasking then are men. It is imperative, therefore, to stick to the topic at hand and stay focused on one point at a time to keep your partner with you during your talk. Reciting a laundry list of concerns will soon cause your partner to tune you out. Make it clear from the beginning what your goal is.

5. Keep your point short and simple. Too much detail and too many extra words will cause him to lose track of the point. Do not keep repeating the same point. And do not dredge up past issues that have nothing to do with the current subject. This will also cause him to stop listening and processing. Make your point once, then stop talking and let him respond.

6. Avoid accusations and use "I" statements. Blaming your partner only causes more separation and defensiveness. Communicate using "I" messages rather than "you" messages. For example, rather than saying, "You never pay attention to me," you could say, "I feel upset because I need/want more attention from you." This allows your partner to better understand how you feel and not become immediately defensive about an accusation.

7. Offer positive encouragement. When your partner feels valued for sharing his feelings and allowing you to express yours, he will be more willing to continue openly communicating. Both of you can make positive statements about how much better it feels to be open and honest. If he brings up a difficult subject, rather than bristling, say, "I'm glad you feel comfortable enough to talk to me about this. Let's see if we can make it work for the two of us."

8. Be aware of nonverbal cues. Your body language and tone of voice can have a significant impact on whether or not your partner will listen to you. If you sit with your arms crossed while you're saying how sorry you are about hurting him, he will "listen" to your constricted, tight body language rather than to your actual apology. This also works in reverse. Women are very gifted at picking up subtle nonverbal cues, which can lead to far more damage than the actual words used.

Couples will find that the benefits of practicing these communication skills will improve your relationship in general, as well as spill over into the bedroom. When a woman feels that her needs are being met, she will feel less anger and resentment, and the door to a more loving and affectionate way of relating to each other will open. If you and your partner are having trouble communicating, seek out a professional, such as a marriage counselor, psychologist, or pastor, who can help you start relating to each other in ways that are healthy and positive. When this is accomplished, a better relationship has a chance to flourish.

Frequently Asked Question...

I like sex, but my husband is a terrible lover. How do I get him to be better without hurting his feelings? As you well know, discussing sexual prowess with your partner can be very intimidating and is like taking a knife to his family jewels. Yet in order for you to be happy with your relationship, emotionally and physically, you should communicate to your partner what it is you want from him. For instance, if during sex he is doing something that you really don't like, show him what it is that you do like and slowly move his hand there. Rather than use full sentences and lots of words, men prefer that women signal pleasure with body movements, groans, and soft moans. Nonverbal feedback is critically important to men—they truly want to please women—but if they feel threatened or criticized in any way, they may become immediately defensive and shut down. Men, as do women, want to feel reassured and accepted. If your partner is trying to "listen" to you through your movements, your subtle guiding hands, and positive feedback, he will feel less threatened and most likely venture to even more adventurous grounds.

Pillow Talk: One of the Most Important Languages You Can Learn

Suppose you and your partner are having sex, but you feel that your sexual needs aren't being met. Perhaps you want more foreplay or kissing. Maybe you need more time to be stimulated before actual sex occurs. Or you want to tell your partner about a particular "spot" that really turns you on. Your partner can't read your mind, and he will naturally assume that all is well if you keep quiet, so you need to communicate your needs to him without putting him on the defensive. Men are particularly sensitive to sexual feedback. Your partner may feel corrected or criticized if you tell him what to do. So, during the actual act of sexual intimacy, it may be best to use fewer words and more bodily hints, like moans and sighs to signify that he is pleasing you. Tell him what you do like and he's guaranteed to do more of it! If your words don't seem to be working, gently take his hand and guide it to the right place. Men take great pride in their ability to please their partners in bed. Keep this in mind: If you're happy—and you've communicated that to him—then he will be happy, too.

Sexual intimacy is an opportunity for honesty, sharing, and closeness, not criticism. Be sure that the tone of your voice conveys what you want, but in a way that you are likely to be heard.

> *"When you are in love, you can't fall asleep because*
> *reality is better than your dreams."*
> —DR. SEUSS

The Bedroom–Libido Connection

So now that you have learned how to communicate more openly, honestly, and effectively using words, what message is your bedroom sending? Is it a place that invites open and intimate communication? Is it conducive to rest and relaxation? Interestingly, how you and your partner decorate your bedroom does in fact influence the quality of your sex life. The ancient Chinese principle of Feng Shui, placing certain objects and structures in a harmonious fashion as well as implementing colors, compass directions, and natural elements like wood, minerals, fire, water, and earth is thought to attract good energy and fortune. You can use these same principles to transform your bedroom into a romantic retreat—a "love shack"!

In order to preserve the bedroom as a sacred place for you and your partner, use it only for sleep and intimacy. Avoid distractions such as computers, work materials, exercise equipment, or television. According to a recent study, "If there's no television in the bedroom, the frequency of sexual intercourse doubles."[1] In addition, certain television programs are far more likely to lessen passion than others. Violent films apparently put a halt on sexual relations for half of all couples, while reality shows decrease passion for one-third. Bottom line: Take the TV out of the bedroom. If you can't, at least stop watching violent shows or reality

TV programs if you want to boost your libido/sexual intimacy.

Whether you are trying to attract a new relationship or lover or are trying to recharge your present relationship, the following tips will help create a romantic refuge, a "hot spot" for love. If you're ready to spice it up a bit more, look into feng shui and personalize it even more!

Paint with sexual colors. Warm colors, such as browns, beiges, reds, apricots, and yellows, are best. Red, the color of love and passion, is best for sexual energy. Yellow is another recommended color, as it symbolizes communication.

Remove excess clutter from the bed. Remove lacy pillows, dolls, and stuffed animals. The bed should be comfortable, without too many accents or an overflow of pillows.

Nightstands. Place a red object on the female nightstand to increase eroticism in the female partner. For the male nightstand, place a something made of copper, such as a jar of copper scraps or a copper sculpture. Copper represents the male essence and enhances eroticism. Or find objects that are stimulating and significant to both of you.

These meaningful changes will allow you and your partner an intimate, relaxing place that belongs only to you. When the message of the room is "leave your stress and anxiety outside," your communication will be guided by love and understanding rather than frustration or resentments.

Shared Time: The Language of Spending Time Together

Time is the most precious commodity each of us gives to another. Withholding it from your partner can signal an end to a relationship. In order for couples to build good communication skills—both inside and outside the bedroom—they need to spend time together. Even if you're not engaged in a deep discussion, just the act of being together is a form of communication. You're saying to each other, "I love to be in your company" and "Being together as a couple is a high priority for me." Start sharing the following lifestyle habits and see how things begin to sizzle in and out of the bedroom:

Have a regular date night. Find a babysitter or call the grandparents so you can go out to dinner. If money's an issue, share a picnic together at the park. Or have lunch together instead of dinner. Go for a stroll or visit a museum.

Go to bed together. How often does one of you watch a movie in the living room while the other reads a book in bed and falls asleep? If you enjoy different activities, this is okay some nights, but it shouldn't be your every day/every night ritual. Find a movie that you can both enjoy, and then go to bed together at the same time.

Eat together. Try to share a meal together at least two or three times a week, if not more. Go even further by lighting some candles, opening a nice bottle of wine, and turning off the TV. Let your partner know that having a special meal together is enjoyable. If you have children, pick a night when you can feed the kids and then have a candlelit dinner together after they go to bed.

Work together on a certain project or goal. It can be as simple as washing the car together or fixing something in the house. Or it can be more ambitious, like painting the living room or building a deck on the house. Accomplishing a goal together is a wonderful bonding experience!

Create a target you're both looking forward to. Those couples who say, "We're both so looking forward to getting away to have some down time together in a couple of weeks," or are in some way looking forward to being together in a special place, "just the two" of them, create an expectation that helps them think and act like a couple who cherish being with one another. It's a language of love that helps them feel bonded to one another, and creates its own brand of intimacy.

Communication is the life-saving bridge between you and your partner. By honestly looking at the level of your present relationship and finding ways to improve your communication skills, you and your partner will reach a higher level of emotional, spiritual, and physical connection. And before you know it, you'll be looking forward to "connecting" under the covers, too!

Communicating with Your Doctor

Having a physician whom you trust and with whom you can freely communicate is key in maintaining optimum health and a strong libido. If you feel embarrassed, rushed, judged, or criticized during your visit, you probably should find a new doctor who has the needed time and compassion to best address your issues. Over the years, I have had many questions asked of me, many of which came from patients who stated they felt too embarrassed to bring them up with other doctors. Here are five ways to best communicate with your doctor during your visit.

- Use your office visit time wisely. Realize that you deserve the time. Your time with your physician is for you—for your health to be assessed and the best treatment to be given. This is your right—not to mention that you are paying for it—so have the courage to express your needs.

- Bring a list of questions with you. Time is of the essence for both you and your physician, so use it in the most productive way possible. I truly appreciate when patients bring in a detailed list so we both know that we have covered all of her concerns.

- View yourself and your physician as partners in your overall health and well-being. It is best to see the relationship in this way—by partnering you are collaborating with one another, communicating honestly and striving to provide the best care for you.

■ Be completely honest and vulnerable—share everything. Over the years, I have had patients who were very timid about asking questions. With enough prompting, I can get them to ask what they really want to ask—not what they "should" be asking. If you can't be completely honest and vulnerable with your gynecologist, then who can you feel comfortable with? And keep in mind that to an OB/GYN, there really is no such thing as an embarrassing question about your sexual health—which includes libido.

■ Don't expect your OB/GYN to read your mind. You have a right to expect a great deal of professionalism from your doctor, but keep in mind that s/he isn't a mind reader. Just as your partner cannot read your mind, neither can your gynecologist. Express what is happening right now. Don't wait for the next visit or delay asking about what you really want to know. When you are taking better care of yourself, you, your partner, and everyone else in your life will benefit.

My goal in this book is to give you the facts and the *permission* to strengthen libido and therefore to help you improve your life. For many women, this attention to libido requires a significant change: a change in their schedules, in their perception of themselves, and in the way they communicate with their partners. Women cannot simply stop the routine of their lives—they have to work, they have to take care of their children, and they have to maintain their homes. But you *must* allow yourself to add to that list: "I must take care of *myself*." Why? Because it's your job to take care of you. You're worth caring for, and you must believe that. When you are satisfied, those around you know it and relate to you more openly and lovingly. Learn to say "no" to those tasks and responsibilities that can be delegated to someone else, and say "yes" to intimacy, self-esteem, and joyfulness. Learn to communicate your concerns and your needs to the most important people in your life: your loved ones, your doctor, and *yourself.*

Questions for Reflection

1. How do you feel about the quality of your relationship? Look back at the list at the beginning of this chapter and write down your answers.

2. What do you feel is lacking in your relationship?

3. How can you best communicate this to your partner?

4. In what specific ways can you and your partner spend more time together? Do you share mutual sport interests? An interest in the arts? Can you do household projects together? Plan more vacations? Schedule more date nights?

5. Have you discussed your sexual health concerns with your doctor?

6. Is there anything that you might be shying away from because you are embarrassed? With your partner? With your doctor?

Resources

Chapter 1

1. Weeks, David J. *Secrets of the Superyoung: The Scientific Reasons Some People Look Ten Years Younger than They Really Are—And Now You Can, Too.* New York: Berkley Books, 1999.

2. Crenshaw, Theresa. *The Alchemy of Love and Lust: Discovering Our Sex Hormones and How They Determine Who We Love, When We Love, and How Often We Love.* New York: Putnam, 1996.

3. Spitz, Rene and Diane Eyer. "Mother-Infant Bonding: A Scientific Fiction." *Human Nature* 5(1): 69–94.

4. The Touch Research Institute at the University of Miami. www.miami.edu/touch-research/research.htm

5. Buss, Jennifer. Kinsey Institute for Research in Sex, Gender, and Reproduction. www.kinseyinstitute.org

6. Gallup, Gordon, G. et al. "Does Semen Have Antidepressant Properties?" *Archives of Sexual Behavior* 31(3) (2002): 289–93.

7. National Heart and Lung Institute (NIH): http://him.nhlbi.nih.gov

8. Farnham, Alan. "Is Sex Necessary?" www.forbes.com/2003/

9. Komisaruk, Barry R. and C. Beyers-Flores, and B. Whipple. *The Science of Orgasm.* Baltimore, MD: The Johns Hopkins University Press, 2006.

10. Ornish, Dean. *Love and Survival: The Scientific Basis for the Healing Power of Intimacy.* New York: Harper Collins, 1998.

Suggested Reading and Resources

Barbach, Loni. *For Yourself: The Fulfillment of Female Sexuality.* New York: Signet, Division of Penguin Books, 2000.

Berman, Laura. *Real Sex for Real Women: Intimacy, Pleasure & Sexual Well-being.* New York: DK Publishing, 2008.

Sex Information and Education Council of the United States. www.siecus.org

Chapter 2

1. Altman, Alan M.D. "Patient Information: Sexual Problems in Women." *UpToDate*.com, 2006.

2. Basson, Roemary. "Using a Different Model for Female Sexual Response to Address Women's Problematic Low Sexual Desire." *Journal of Sex and Marital Therapy* 27 (2001): 395–403.

3. Leibovich, Lori. "Danger: Low Voltage," *Cookie*, October 2008, 96–106.

4. Cox, John L. et al. "Detection of Postnatal Depression. Development of the 10-item Edinburgh Postnatal Depression Scale." *The British Journal of Psychiatry* 150 (1987): 782–86.

5. *Glamour*, February 2009.

Suggested Reading
Davis, Michele Weiner. *The Sex-Starved Marriage: Boosting Your Marriage Libido; A Couple's Guide*. New York: Simon & Schuster, 2003.

Hendrix, Harville, and Helen LaKelly Hunt. *Getting the Love You Want.* New York: Henry Holt and Company, 2007.

Masters, William. H., and Virginia. E. Johnson. *Human Sexual Response*. Boston: Little, Brown, 1966.

Northrup, Christiane. *Women's Bodies, Women's Wisdom.* New York: Bantam Books, 2006.

Chapter 3

1. P. Koch, et al. "'Feeling Frumpy': The Relationships Between Body Image and Sexual Response Changes in Midlife Women." *The Journal of Sex Research*, November 2005

2. Heldman, Caroline. "Out-of-Body Image: Women See Themselves Through Eyes of Others." *Ms. Magazine*, Spring issue, 2008.

Suggested Reading and Resources
Brandon, Nathaniel. *How to Raise Your Self-Esteem: The Proven Action-Oriented Approach to Greater Self-Respect and Self-Confidence.* New York: Bantam Books, 1987.
Martin, Courtney. *Perfect Girls, Starving Daughters: The Frightening New Normalcy of Hating Your Body.* New York: The Free Press, 2007.

Weiner, Jessica. *Life Doesn't Begin 5 Pounds From Now.* New York: Simon Spotlight Entertainment, imprint of Simon & Schuster, 2006.

Chapter 4

1. Geary, David C. *Male, Female: The Evolution of Human Sex Differences.* Washington, D.C.: American Psychological Association Publisher, 1998.

2. Josanovic, Hristina, J. Lundberg, P. Karlsson, A. Cerin, T. Saijo, A. Varrone, C. Halldin, and A. Nordström. "Sex Differences in the Serotonin 1A Receptor and Serotonin Transporter Binding in the Human Brain Measured by PET." *NeuroImage* 39(3) (February 2008), 1408–19.

3. Baron-Cohen, Simon. *The Essential Difference. The Truth about the Male and Female Brain.* New York: Basic Books/Perseus Books Group, 2003.

4. Pease, Barbara, and Allan Pease. *Why Men Don't Have a Clue and Women Always Need More Shoes: The Ultimate Guide to the Opposite Sex.* New York: Broadway Books, 2004.

5. Trivers, Robert. "Parental Investment and Sexual Selection." In F. B. G. Campbell. *Sexual Selection and the Descent of Man.* London: Heinemann Educational, 1972, 136–39.

Suggested Reading and Resources
Amen, Daniel G., M.D. *Sex on the Brain: 12 Lessons to Enhance Your Love Life.* New York: Harmony Books, 2007.

Becker, Jill B. (Ed.). *Sex Differences in the Brain: From Genes to Behavior.* New York: Oxford University Press, 2007.

Blum, Deborah. *Sex on the Brain: The Biological Differences Between Men and Women.* New York: Penguin, 1998.

Legato, Marianne J., M.D. *Why Men Never Remember and Women Never Forget.* Emmaus, PA: Rodale Books, 2006.

Pease, Barbara, and Allan Pease. *Why Men Don't Have a Clue and Women Always Need More Shoes: The Ultimate Guide to the Opposite Sex.* New York: Broadway Books, 2004.

Pease, Barbara, and Allan Pease. *Why Men Don't Listen and Women Can't Read Maps: How We're Different and What to Do About It.* New York: Broadway Books, 2001.

Singh, Devendra. "Female Mate Value at a Glance: Relationship of Waist-to-Hip Ratio to Health, Fecundity and Attractiveness." *Neuroendocrinology Letters* 23, Suppl. 4 (2002): 81–91.

Chapter 5

1. Durex Global Sex Survey, 2007/2008. www.durexworld.com/en-US/SexualWellbeingSurvey/

2. Wyatt, Tristam D. *Pheromones and Animal Behaviour: Communication by Smell and Taste.* Oxford: Cambridge University Press, 2003. University of Oxford.

3. Frobose, Gabriele, et al. *Lust and Love: Is It More than Chemistry?* Cambridge: Royal Society of Chemistry, 2006.

4. Stern, Kathleen, and M. K. McClintock. "Regulation of Ovulation by Human Pheromones." *Nature* 392 (March 12, 1998): 177.

5. Hirsch, Alan, M.D. www.scienceofsmell.com

Suggested Reading and Resources
Recipes for Love from Celebrity Chefs and Cookbook Authors. www.starchefs.com/features/aphrodisiacs/volume_02/html

Cooking with Aphrodisiacs. www.vat19.com/dvds/cwa.cfm

Collection of articles and essays on aphrodisiacs. www.aphrodisiology.com/

Aphrodisiac Recipes & Food Links.
  www.gourmetsleuth.com/recipes_aphro.asp

Chapter 6

1. National Consumer League, 2003. www.nclnet.org/research/6/26/03

2. Roizen, Michael, and Mehmet Oz. *Reader's Digest,* April 2007: 49.

3. American Psychological Association, 2005. www.apa.org

4. Meyer, David, et al. www.apa.org/journals/xhp/press_releases/august_2001/
  xhp274763.html.

5. Porges, Stephen. www.stephenporges.info

6. Taylor, Shelley E., L. C. Klein, B. P. Lewis, T. L. Gruenewald, R. A. R. Gurung,
  and J. A. Updegraff. "Female Responses to Stress: Tend and Befriend, Not Fight
  or Flight." *Psychological Review* 107 (3) (2000), 41–429.

7. Carter, C. Sue, et al www.apa.org/monitor/fcb08/oxytocin.html

8. Holmes, Thomas and Richard Rahe, 1967. "The Social Readjustment Rating
  Scale." *Journal of Psychosomatic Research* 11(2): 213–19.

9. Carmichael, Mary. "Who Says Stress Is Bad for You?" *Newsweek,* February 23,
  2009.

Helpful Resources for Stress Management
Ways to identify and manage stress effectively: www.stress.org

Helpguide: www.helpguide.org/mental/stress

Research causes, symptoms, and treatments of stress: www.healthline.com

Effective ways to reduce stress: www.aiht.edu

Essential health information for women and stress:
  www.ivillage.com/mindbody/mbstress/topics

Coping with stress: www.copingtoday.com/coping-with-stress/links.htm

Calculating Your Stress Quotient
Holmes and Rahe Stress Test: www.stress-management.net/stress-test.htm

Specific Relaxation/Meditation Resources
Progressive muscle relaxation: www.guidetopsychlogy.com/pmr.htm and
   www.medicinenet.com

Virtual meditation slide show: www.selfhelpmagazine.com/articles/stress

Information regarding craniosacral therapy: www.craniosacraltherapy.org

Craniosacral information: www.northshoreacupuncture.com

Behrends, Vicki RCST, HHP, MA. Interviews, 2008-2009. victoria.bcst@gmail.com

Resources on healing therapies: www.wellnessinstitute.net

Healing from trauma: www.traumahealing.com

Information regarding polyvagal theory: www.wikipedia.org/wiki/Stephen_Porges

Chapter 7

1. Nurnberg, H George, et al. *Sildenafil Treatment of Women with Antidepressant-As-sociated Sexual Dysfunction.* JAMA. 2008 Jul 23;300(4):395-404

2. Shifren, Jan L., et al. (2000). "Transdermal Testosterone Treatment in Women with Impaired Sexual Function after Oophorectomy. *New England Journal of Medicine,* 343: 682–88.

3. Davis, Susan R., et al.,(2008). Testosterone for Low Libido in Postmeno-pausal Women Not Taking Estrogen. *New England Journal of Medicine:* 359 (19) 2005–2017.

Suggested Reading and Resources
Diagnostic and Statistical Manual of Mental Disorders, 4th Edition, Text Revision. Washington, DC: American Psychiatric Association, 2000. www.psych.org

Rosen, Raymond. "The Female Sexual Function Index (FSFI): A Multidimensional Self-Report Instrument for the Assessment of Female Sexual Function." *Journal of Sex and Marital Therapy* 26(2) (2000):191–208.

DeRogatis, Leonard, et al. "The Female Sexual Distress Scale-Revised (FSDS-R): Validation of the Female Sexual Distress Scale—Revised for Assessing Distress in Women with Hypoactive Sexual Desire Disorder. *Journal of Sexual Medicine* 5(2) (2007): 357–64.

To find sex therapists or counselors
American Association of Sexuality Educators, Counselors, and Therapists. www.aasect.org

Chapter 8

1. Fisher, Helen. *Why We Love: The Nature and Chemistry of Romantic Love*. New York: Henry Holt, 2004.

2. Panzer, Claudia, et al. *Journal of Sexual Medicine*, 3(1) (2006): 104–112.

3. Rossouw, Jacques F., et al. *Journal of American Medical Association*, 288(3) (2002): 321-333.

4. Gazzaruso, Carmine, et al. *Journal of the American College of Cardiology, 51(21):* 2040-4, 2008.

5. Troxel, Wendy, et al. SLEEP 2009, 23rd Annual Meeting of Associated Professional Sleep Societies, Abstract, June 10, 2009.

Helpful Websites
American Diabetes Association: www.diabetes.org

National Sleep Foundation—sleep hygiene and sleep disorders: www.sleepfoundation.org

Centers for Disease Control and Prevention—sleep and health conditions: www.cdcinfo@cdc.gov

Chapter 9

1. Salomoni, Serenella. *The New York Times,* January 16, 2006. "Television in Bedroom Halves Your Sex Life."

Suggested Reading

Chapman, Gary. *The Five Love Languages: How to Express Heartfelt Commitment to Your Mate.* Chicago: Northfield Publishing Company, 2004.

Gray, John, Ph.D. *Mars and Venus in the Bedroom: A Guide to Lasting Romance and Passion.* New York: HarperCollins, 1995.

Schnarch, David. *Passionate Marriage: Keeping Love & Intimacy Alive in Committed Relationships.* New York: Henry Holt and Company, 1997.

Weiner Davis, Michele. *The Sex-Starved Marriage: Boosting Your Marriage Libido, A Couple's Guide.* New York: Simon & Schuster, 2003.

INDEX

ABOUT THE AUTHOR

Diana E. Hoppe, M.D., F.A.C.O.G., is a highly respected, board-certified obstetrician/gynecologist in private practice in San Diego, California. She is co-founder of her private group practice, Pacific Coast Women's Health, Inc., and medical director/principal investigator of Pacific Coast Research Center in Encinitas, California, a medical research center that conducts international clinical research trials in the field of women's health, including menopause, perimenopause, and libido. Presently, she is a primary investigator involved in an international clinical trial for a new medication to treat hypoactive female sexual desire disorder. Dr. Hoppe's unique combination of qualifications—she is conducting clinical trials with pharmaceutical companies as a scientific investigator and as a compassionate, concerned obstetrician/gynecologist—places her at the heart of the issue of improving women's sexual lives. Enabling women to reap valuable knowledge from her research and years of clinical practice will free them from the chains that have bound them to ignore their desire to thrive—not only in the sexual arena, but in *all* aspects of their lives.

Dr. Hoppe is also a national and international speaker and published author of clinical trials in the field of women's health, and is actively involved in establishing women's rights through the American College of Obstetricians and Gynecologists and the House of Delegates with the California Medical Association. She has frequently appeared on both national and local television, highlighting research on women's health, specifically on women's libido and its effect on overall well-being.

To contact the author, write to:
Diana Hoppe, M.D.
Pacific Coast Women's Health
317 N. El Camino Real, Suite 306
Encinitas, CA 92024

www.DrDianaHoppe.com